Life in Speech

Rebecca Wuest, M.A., CCC-SLP

For my children, Jamie, Alex, and Ana, with love.

ACKNOWLEDGMENTS

I am very grateful to all the incredible speech-language pathologists who entrusted me with their stories.

Note from the Author

I began my career in 1993 as a speech-language pathologist (SLP) working with brain injury survivors at The Rehabilitation Institute of Chicago. In 2019, I joined the ranks of these survivors when I was struck by a tanker truck while on the interstate on my way to work.

 It was immediately apparent to me after the accident, even with my muddled mind, that I had suffered a significant brain injury. I couldn't tolerate light, or noise, and spent my days alone in my quiet, darkened bedroom. But worse than the constant throbbing headache, imbalance, double vision, or tinnitus, was the painful awareness that I couldn't remember a conversation from earlier in the day, or solve a simple daily problem, or come up with the words that I needed to clearly express myself.

At first, I resisted when my doctor recommended speech therapy. I didn't want anyone else to see how badly I'd been impacted by the TBI and was especially worried about my cognitive status. However, there was no way to conceal my deficits when early in the therapy process, I was asked to solve the Zoo Puzzle, a fairly basic logic/planning task. I knew I should be able to complete it, that it should be easy for me. The realization that I couldn't make sense of it at all completely panicked me. Scared and defeated, I put my head down on the therapy table and sobbed.

Slowly, however, I began to improve, conquered that damned Zoo Puzzle, started to drive again, and went back to work part-time. I am profoundly grateful to my SLP, who skillfully and patiently guided me through the tedious process (I'm sure for her as well as me) of recovery. She convinced me that I could make gains, and never let me give up on myself.

Having known struggle and frustration, achievement and reward, on both sides of the therapy table, I want to share with you the lived experiences of other SLPs as they work with individuals in the varied aspects of our field. I'm extremely proud to be able to call them my colleagues.

Life in Speech Therapy

Who's Gonna Stay?

RW: What made you become an SLP? What drew you to the field?

SLP: I like to say naivete, and truly, when I got into this it was naive. My dream job when I was 18 years old, and unaware of the world, was to go to each country and learn their language and their culture, and then get moved to the next one, and somehow get paid millions. Then I took a linguistics class, and they talked about how the work of linguistics is so underpaid. So it was a pipe dream.

But speech pathology really was something, and I had so much background with kids with special needs. The more I learned about speech pathology, I just thought that was the coolest thing, and I felt like it was such a gift. I love to talk. It's my big hobby, and to be able to participate in giving that to someone else's life, to me it was the ultimately coolest dream, the coolest job. Then once I started classwork, I loved it. It was an excellent fit, and the rest is history.

RW: What about your work has frustrated you?

SLP: I do want to say that patient care has almost never frustrated me. There was a time when I would come home and talk about how much I loved this job, and all the really cool things that I saw, and the patient victories that I was in. It just was so neat, so I don't recall the time I've ever come home, with rare exception, and complained about doing evaluations. I don't think I've even complained about paperwork. I like the paperwork process. For me, all of my complaints regarding our career are simply summed up in the current system and state of health care and the pay.

Also it's incredibly expensive to be in this career with as many certifications as I have, and that you need. I feel like I get nickeled and dimed, and that's probably a petty complaint in the long run, but that irritates me as a provider. I wouldn't mind paying ASHA [American Speech-Language-Hearing Association] if they did more for us. I get, for instance, very annoyed that anytime I want transgender voice handouts, well that's $45. If I'd like to do LSVT [Lee Silverman Voice Treatment] Loud, that's $1000, and now everybody's moving to SPEAK OUT!, so you're either writing grants to get that education covered, or that's another $1500. Then to maintain that every year, it's another $50, so it's just I find that the nickel and diming is really annoying.

RW: Absolutely. I think that ASHA kind of owes us at least free handouts.

SLP: This is funny, and coming from a world where I work really closely with the ENTs: the last group of surgeons I worked for, they would invite me to all of their sponsored events. Speech is lucky when we get a coffee when our vendors come in, and they're like, "Oh, I'm gonna bring you coffee, or Panera." These dudes are eating Surf and Turf for free with an open bar! I would imagine it's at least seven grand that these vendors shell out, just to talk to our surgeons about surgical products, and they sponsor our journal clubs for ENTs. And it's unlimited, so I come too. I'm not buying surgical equipment, but these vendors have to shut up and pay for me and whatever I want, because I rolled up with the big guys. I mean, the residents [doctors in training] will get two Surf and

Turfs: one to eat there and one to take home, and there's no shame in it. They bring it in from the nicest restaurants in town.

RW: What keeps you going in your career at this point?

SLP: Sadly, it's nothing, because I'm actively quitting my career. The systematic frustrations are so prolific, and so disruptive. I actively worry about an active shooter situation, and sometimes it's hard for me to go to sleep. It's such a horribly abusive environment being in healthcare now, between the staff and the patients, that I genuinely worry in an institution as large as mine that somebody's going to open fire. With that said, I've been in two active shooter threats in my six-year career, so it's not like it's an unrealistic possibility. I mean, violence against healthcare workers is only increasing, because we don't have the staff. We can't meet their needs and the patients' frustration is just boiling over.

Imagine if you take that crazy person in a car who you cut off, so they fly by you and give you the finger, right? Now you put them in a stressful medical situation where they might not have hope. I mean, the hospital is full of those people. I was just assaulted for the first time by a patient because he was mad that I couldn't take him to the bathroom on hip precautions. Then on top of that, I got a little bit, not a ton, but I did get a little bit of kickback when I said I wanted to report this, because of who this patient was.

I also worry about hurting a patient and going to jail. You know, there've been cases of nurses who have been under stressful situations, and given the wrong doses of medication. For speech, it's not that I'm gonna literally kill someone, but I sure may end up in court one day over something that happened to somebody because I didn't have enough support. God forbid, somebody falls in my session, you know? I worry more and more about the litigious aspect. At the end of the day, if we were helping people, I think I would stay. I am barely paying my bills, and thank God, I am paying my bills, but only because I'm financially very savvy. Why did I work seven years for a career to barely pay my bills, get assaulted at my job, and not see good patient outcomes, because we're not seeing good patient outcomes anymore.

RW: Are you okay? Were you injured?

SLP: No, I had no physical injuries. I just surprised myself and I think it surprised the patient, because I instantly stepped back and threw my finger up and was like, you're not doing this, you get your hands off me. It was an immediate defense, and it was a very strong reaction. It was nipped in the bud very quickly, and from what I understand they didn't give anyone else a hard time, so that's good.

RW: Was the patient cognitively intact?

SLP: Yeah, they were cognitively intact, and they shoved me because they needed to go to the bathroom. They needed to have a bowel movement. There was no one to take them, and so the staff was encouraging the patient to defecate themself, so that they didn't have to wait. They found that very compromising, as I would too. But that doesn't mean that I can ambulate somebody on hip precautions. So that's truly the state of where healthcare is. It's like just please poop and pee yourself in your diaper, because we have nobody to help you right now, and we'll come get it later. We'll change your diaper with the door wide open because nobody seems to care about dignity anymore. So, It's horrible. Not closing the door, I find at the very least not excusable. I think patients using their diapers have just sprung out of the fact that we have no staff to meet these needs, so how are you gonna do it?

RW: The indignity of that is just tragic.

SLP: It's shocking.

RW: I think you were also exposed to smoke at work?

SLP: Yeah, so the first institution I worked at was in the middle of a rural area. It was a nursing home and there was an active fire in the ceiling. I mean, this was within probably three months of me starting at work. I had to transport patients to different areas to get away from the smoke from the fire. We were all rushing to get them out. I had no idea what I was doing, and I ended up with pneumonia from what they speculated was smoke inhalation. It's not like it was pouring into my lungs, but it was just being around the smoke for that long. Then my employer really didn't want me to take off for pneumonia. It was a battle with them.

The one thing I've learned about healthcare that just really upsets me too, is that they don't care about the health of their employees. I mean, that's very evident to me. I've had smoke inhalation. I've been assaulted by a patient, and in two active shooter threats. I've also had an HIV exposure that I was on workers comp for.

I almost ended up in a lawsuit, because they didn't want to pay for safety equipment. They didn't see it as safety equipment for me, as a speech pathologist, but that's what it was; they didn't want to carry the right voice prosthetics in stock. If you pull out an old prosthetic, and a patient's leaking gastric contents into their airway, you have to have something to plug that up. I was in the OR with the ENT for two hours to resolve that. Even though I had my safety glasses on, there was so much coughing and so much blood that my glasses were fogged. When I was trying to see if we had the solution, I lifted my glasses just to peek, and fluids came right into my eye. I was blamed for that. I had to consult with a lawyer. It was so horrible. I just worry about my health at this job.

RW: May I ask if you were infected?

SLP: No, thank God. Ironically, the week that I settled my workers comp and got my last negative HIV result, I was assaulted by the patient and I was like, I can't even, this is ridiculous.

RW: I can't imagine how stressful that must have been, waiting for the HIV results.

SLP: It was very stressful because they didn't want to pay for any of the testing and they legally had to. It was a huge battle back and forth, because it was a lot of money on their end. Thankfully this particular patient was very medically compliant, so I knew that their levels were undetectable. The idea that I could get HIV was very low. However, they were supposed to also test for hep [hepatitis] B and hep C, which I have no immunity to, despite several rounds of vaccinations. I'm just not immune. They kept running the wrong labs on the patient, so the patient eventually refused to keep coming back. We never knew about the hep B or C status. But in my mind, I was also thinking, What are the odds that this patient's raging with Hep B and C and is compliant with HIV meds? I thought this was low risk, but it was a whole year to be sure. At the time, I was selling plasma to pay off my car, because the hourly rate to sell plasma was so much higher than the PRN [work as needed] rate. It took away some of my income, because when I was on HIV precautions I couldn't donate.

RW: Everything about that is awful. But to think that you are selling plasma because it was more money than the PRN rate for SLP work!

SLP: By a long shot. It was like $70 for 45 minutes. I do believe in certain areas that you could make $70 PRN, but my state was not one of them. But $70 for 45 minutes of time where you do nothing, and you don't have paperwork, and you don't have to be exposed to threats. It was easy.

RW: I'm so sorry for what you've been through. I can't even get my head around it all. I'm just amazed to see you still smiling.

SLP: I'm smiling because I have an exit plan, and that makes me so sad.

RW: I'm sure it's bittersweet.

SLP: It is.

RW: Hopefully things will change in the field. If enough people do what you're doing, and say "No, I'm not going to do this under these circumstances," eventually there'll be such a need for SLPs that they're gonna have to give us what we need to have a decent quality of life.

SLP: Well my frustration comes from that, even with the safety equipment and stuff, as soon as something adverse happens, and now they're in hot water, it changes. They don't listen to us prophylactically. They don't listen to the things that we need to do our job. I do think some of that stems from the fact that speech is often not in leadership positions within rehab. The other thing is that we're such a poorly understood profession that when I say, "I need these plugs for this patient's neck, it's for his safety and mine," they don't look at that until something bad happens. We had to send that patient back to surgery.

Maybe you should have listened to your advanced-degree clinical professional.

RW: I think you've talked a little bit about what you have found rewarding, and it sounds like it was the patients.

SLP: Yeah, I do love the patients. I still think as far as hands-on patient care, that this career is a 10 out of 10 for me. I think it's an excellent fit, especially as hard as I've worked to get into working in cancer. You probably know, working in cancers, it's tough. Not every SLP's cut out for it. Not every SLP has access to that education, and I just kind of got into it by a fluke, but it's been a tremendously good fit for me. I still just love the career. I love helping people intimately through some of the worst times of their life, and sometimes that includes helping them die. There's a lot of reward in that if your mindset is correct.

RW: Right. A good death.

SLP: A good death, you're achieving what you want to achieve. For example, tricks to help patients communicate throughout the end. I had one family I worked really closely with, and when the patient passed I went to the funeral. I had never heard his voice before because when he came to me, he was aphonic [without voice]. At the funeral I asked the family, Is there any way I can listen to his voice? And they said "Yes," and they played it. This man had the deepest southern twang I had ever heard, and I just started laughing because I didn't picture him like that.

This patient ended up writing a book about his life by answering questions like, "What's something you remember from your childhood?" Everything that he shared was written, because he couldn't talk. His family said, "You know, all of his thoughts for the last six months are on paper. We saved all this, we have all of this writing, and we found out what a blessing that is. We have these boxes of notebooks, and we're gonna have them published." It's a really beautiful thing, because he was able to have hope up until the end. He was able to make progress and remain calm through his aphonic diagnosis. There's a lot of really great things that came out of therapy, even though I think a lot of people would consider it a failure that he ultimately passed away. But the goal was never to cure him. The goal was to get him through with dignity and being able to communicate, and figure out how he could still taste soda. Again, we found ways to do that.

RW: I feel so sad that you're leaving the field, but I support your decision to take care of yourself. I completely support you, but I think it's a tremendous loss for the field.

SLP: I really appreciate that, because it's hard, and it's bad. One of the things that I was thinking about is that I had a hundred CEUs [continuing education units] of education in three years. It was an absurd amount of education when I got into cancer because I had no idea what I was doing. I had to learn all this stuff, and then all of a sudden you're an expert, and you're a specialist. You're so sought after, then only to realize that it still didn't have any impact on the say I had in my pay, or my benefits, or my time off. The fact is that these institutions that work with cancer patients are huge, and they don't have to, so they're not going to produce any type of flexibility for their employees.

It would have been much more advantageous for me to take that thousand dollars spent on CEUs and go get Botox, and extensions, and breast implants, and go seek out a husband. At least I would have increased my income by a hundred percent, maybe more. Maybe if it's really good injections, I think I could get myself a sugar daddy. That would have been more advantageous financially for me than investing in continuing education to help cancer patients.

RW: What do you think needs to change in our field? How do we go about doing that?

SLP: First and foremost, one of the things that really frustrates me about this career that needs to change is that speech has a very bully mentality. It's from the time you enter school, through the time you become a professional. You know nurses are known for "eating their young," but that's what we do, too. I mean I hear my colleagues crap on SNF [skilled nursing facility] SLPs all the time, like, "Oh well, they're not gonna get good care because they're going to a SNF SLP."

How are we going to ask for better rights for ourselves when we don't even believe in the person who's our colleague working next to us? There's a lot of strong opinions in speech, and some of them are very unfounded, and some of them are just the bully mentality, and it has to change. It is ridiculous that we don't think we have something to learn from the person next to us. I don't like that at all. So within ourselves, we have to change something. We all have such a hard time unifying, and when we put each other down it does nothing to advance our cause. That's the first thing.

The second thing is, I don't know what the perfect health care solution is, I don't have a degree in any of that, but the system in the United States is just going to have to change. There's probably some middle ground between solely for-profit and solely not-for-profit. But a lot of these not-for-profit institutions like the one I work at are running on for-profit motives, and they're underpaying their workers. They're creating these conditions that are leading to abuse of staff and abusive patients. That definitely has to change as well. We have to be able to get some type of worker's rights for speech therapy, so I guess I'll dive into my project here.

RW: Please do.

SLP: I'm part of an anonymous group of speech therapists that get together over the internet and discuss ways that we can create union solutions for speech therapy. Speech therapy, unlike nursing, does not have any legal grounds independently to unionize, because we don't have enough workers with common interests. A national union is certainly off the table because that would mean trying to unionize on a state level, or on an independent employer level. When SLPs make up only twelve people in an entire hospital system, it's just not enough power. It's never going to happen.

We created this petition to try and ask ASHA to advocate for us in a better way. We felt that ASHA is not doing enough to help us, and that our petition would likely be ignored, which it subsequently was. Right now we're just laying the groundwork, and the paper trail, to ask for help, and hopefully it works. The goal is that they respond and we put this to rest. But they're not doing that right now, because they have too much power and they don't have to, even though we're all technically unified under their certification.

Our next step is to try and rally some PTs [physical therapists] and OTs [occupational therapists] and work with labor lawyers and union organizations to create legislation, or a bill, or to reach politicians. They might be able to put things in place for us such as productivity caps, and enforce laws that already exist that these therapy companies are getting away with exploiting. Not paying us for documentation review, that shouldn't be legal, having us clock out in between patients whenever a patient doesn't show up, that shouldn't be legal, you're at work. But these companies get away with it, and we need a crackdown on that. The productivity caps need to come down for patient safety, and again, patient outcomes, and for our safety as well. As much emphasis as there is on patient safety, there's not nearly as much emphasis on worker safety, and this has become a huge issue in today's climate.

RW: Anything else you want to add?

SLP: I think the biggest thing for me is that it's a career I fell in love with, and it makes me angry that I worked a minimum of seven years to get here, and had to take out a master degree on a debt. I've no protection to recoup any of that lost income. At this point, I'm faced with not retiring in the field. Seriously, we're leaving, and who's gonna stay? We need to elevate the idea that we have a secondary income because we're married, and we have husbands with insurance [the majority of SLPs are female]. If we're getting advanced degrees, we need to be paid. It's got to start with speech therapy. If we're not speaking out for ourselves, if we're not doing anything to help ourselves, it's just not going to advance. It's uncomfortable, but no change ever comes comfortably.

In a Heartbeat

RW: What drew you to the field of speech-language pathology?

SLP: When I was in eighth grade, so about 14 years old, my mother had a CVA [stroke]. I had a sister who was a year older, and we as a family pulled together and really supported, and were involved with, my mom's rehabilitation. She did make a wonderful recovery, but a good part of the next year involved a lot of team kinds of things. This of course was in the early 60s, so these were not the kinds of teams that have been a part of my professional career. There was a woman who was a speech-language pathologist, although it wasn't called that then, she was called a "speech therapist," and I spent a lot of time sitting in the room listening to that exchange. That, I think, was my incentive to pursue a career in a similar field.

RW: I'm glad your mother had a good recovery. What do you think you might have become if not a speech pathologist?

SLP: It's interesting, the way I came into the speech field. I was a Peace Corps volunteer in Ethiopia and I first of all was assigned to a Sudanese refugee camp. My duty was to teach English as a second language to women. As far as we knew, they were the only women from Sudan who were receiving any kind of education whatsoever. I was then sent into Addis Ababa, which was the capital of Ethiopia, and assigned to a job training center where we were teaching English as a second language. We were preparing Ethiopian folks for employment in a new Hilton Hotel that was opening. It was a very interesting assignment, and I have always said they taught me way more than I ever taught them. It was a

16

fascinating part of my early twenties, and really a marvelous experience.

When I finished with the Peace Corp I returned to start my master's degree in speech-language pathology, and subsequently graduated in 1971. I felt like I had had such a rich, interesting amount of experience and exposure prior to coming to graduate school, that it made that experience a whole lot more meaningful. I think it made me a better therapist.

RW: That's a remarkable story. In terms of the field itself, is there anything that you have found frustrating?

SLP: In recent years I've worked in so many different settings. In my most recent setting I was working on a program with the school district in a cluster of their schools. It was called the LEAP program, an early enrichment program for children who were bilingual. Again, that element of being involved with kiddos for whom English was not their first language. So many of my counterparts were at that time kind of fresh out of graduate school, and they were so quick to go to tablets and computers rather than first have any notion of what kind of learner these children were. I think it's foolish to think that every individual learns in the same way. By that time in my experience, having worked in private practice, and a developmental preschool program, as well as with adults, and having experienced just a myriad of things, I knew that there was not the answer in an iPad. So many of them felt that was the end all be all. I felt really frustrated, both in my role with my school, and with my kiddos, trying to be kind of collegial and work as a group, when they thought every solution was on their iPad.

RW: What's kept you going? So many of our younger therapists are leaving the field.

SLP: Well, variety was certainly an incentive for me. Because of my husband's occupation we moved a lot. I worked in a small community where I ended up being in private practice with a physician for 11 years. That physician had a contract to do the physicals for the Union Pacific Railroad. My job was to test the hearing of these folks that worked for the railroad, and it was so much more than just testing their hearing and doing that on an annual basis. If they were in a noisy situation, I would then offer to talk to their supervisor, the safety director for the railroad, about hearing protection and hearing conservation.

No matter what I did, I seemed to be able to move it to another level that would make not only my job more interesting, but add another important element. I for a long time worked with a developmental program. I wrote the grant to begin the first developmental preschool for institutionally based handicapped individuals in my state. That was a wonderful experience. Up until that time, there was a state institution near me, where from the time a child was identified at birth, they put them in the institution. Well, by the late 60s and early 70s, of course, everyone knew that that was not a good idea. The community-based program began to be a really big deal, and I was on the cutting edge of developing and implementing those community-based programs. I also spent 12 years on the state Board of Medicine, as a non-physician member, that licensed and disciplined docs. I got a real opportunity to know physicians throughout the state, and I think to be a real part of that medical piece too.

RW: What did you find most rewarding about your work?

SLP: I think the feedback from the individuals, and also that unspoken celebration when someone gets something. I was working with stroke patients, and I had a woman whose husband deemed me a "swallowologist." It seemed that she was never going to get beyond swallowing ice chips, but she did. Having those kinds of successes. The same thing with children who were severely hearing impaired, to unleash that once they had either amplification or whether it was sign language or whatever; to get that element of communication so that others were able to share and understand. I think in all the settings that I worked, there was always that element of that aha moment for clients, whether they were tall or small. That just was my reward way beyond the paycheck.

RW: Is there anything that you would like to see changed in our field? Anything that you think we need to do differently?

SLP: I remember dealing with ASHA when I was working with foreign accent reduction therapy. It seemed that there was this rigidity and this insensitivity starting at ASHA and filtering down, and I think that was a pretty pervasive frustration that I had. But fortunately, I didn't let it thwart me or stop me. I was able to smile and diplomatically step around it, but I think that was one of the major frustrations.

RW: Do you have a favorite story?

SLP: I remember when I was working in an elementary program and I think I was administering some standardized test, and one of the types of questions was, "How is this, like the other?" The particular question was, "How are a pound and a yard the same?" This little guy looked at me and said, "You can keep a dog in both of them." And I looked at my answer sheet, and I thought, that answer is not there, but he's right! I certainly had delightful, funny times. I think that one of the things that was always the link with my success with my clients was the ability to enjoy and laugh, and not take ourselves so terribly seriously.

RW: You have had a huge amount of experience as an SLP. What would you say to people entering the field or beginning their careers?

SLP: To branch out and not let themselves get pigeonholed, I think. So often folks do. I think that they need to make sure that they try a lot of different age range groups, you know? I know that that was a luxury I had, and perhaps everyone does not. The other thing that I see my younger colleagues doing is embracing the fact that there are now licensed SLPAs [assistants] available, so not to let themselves let those assistants have all the pleasure, and the SLPs get stuck with doing all the assessment and all the reports. I think when they let the assistants do all of the intervention, they're really missing out on a huge piece that can bring such pleasure and joy.

RW: Would you do it all again? Any regrets?

SLP: I would do it all again, in a heartbeat. I have no regrets whatsoever. I have had such a marvelous career.

It's Not the Algebra

RW: So, why did you become a speech therapist? What drew you to the field?

SLP: My path is kind of different because I was actually a pharmacist first. I still have my license for that. I tell my husband, it's my expensive hobby to do pharmacy continuing education! I guess I just wanted a job that didn't have so many nights and holidays and weekends, and also where you had more control over your day-to-day work. In pharmacy you were kind of between the patient and the doctor a lot, and it was people just coming in and out a lot. I wanted to do something different. I was interested in healthcare because my mom actually had a stroke in her forties, and had to learn how to talk again. She's in her eighties now, so she's a trooper, she's a survivor. Seeing the kind of support in healthcare she got, that was definitely part of why I was interested in the field too.

So when I was doing one of my pharmacy rotations, I went around the hospital and observed every job in the hospital, and I thought, Oh this looks better, I would like to do this. Weirdly, I had to take some leveling classes to be able to apply to graduate school. And honestly, pharmacy school was probably harder, but speech pathology grad school was probably harder to get into. They just didn't have as many spaces, but since my story was kind of weird, I think they let me in. They probably wanted a different perspective.

I thought I would work in healthcare, but when I graduated, there weren't very many healthcare jobs. I had just done the school rotation. I was like, Oh well, it was nice to have a school schedule. I'll just do that for a while, but then I ended up really liking it.

RW: In terms of the field, what frustrates you?

SLP: The special education paperwork and the large caseload numbers, that's just the part that gets you down. I should have done work today, which is my day off, because that's my time to do the paperwork for the next week. I don't have time to do it at work.

RW: What keeps you going anyway?

SLP: I really like the students. I like the staff, and I even like the parents. I really like the job itself, and helping the kids learn to be communicators and working on teams at school to help kids do better. For example, when it's a child that might need speech, and special education, and OT [occupational therapy], and you're problem solving as part of a team. Also, I like having longer-term relationships with the kids. Most of my sixth graders I've been with for seven years. I would say the relationships, and just the value behind communication making everybody's life better. At the end of the day, I'm not discounting the algebra teacher, but what is gonna help you better in life? Is it all the time you spent learning algebra, or is it the time you learn how to communicate and talk? Where are you gonna find joy in life? It's gonna be communicating with others.

RW: So true. So what do you think needs to change in our field?

SLP: I think that in our public school district, our staff is somewhat diverse, at least racially. But as a whole, I don't think the field is that diverse. I think there's some growth to do there, because I think men care about communication, and people of all ethnic backgrounds care about communication.

RW: What advice do you have for someone entering the field?

SLP: I do often tell people, don't necessarily get the communication sciences and disorders undergraduate degree. Get an education degree, or maybe a generic communications degree or something like that. Then they could get a job in something else if graduate school doesn't work out. One of my friends at work, her daughter was going to college, and this girl loved math, but she somehow had in her mind she wanted to be a speech therapist. I was like, well, why doesn't she just be a math major, and take a bunch of communication sciences disorders classes as her minor? Just look up three schools and see what their requirements are, and make sure she has those classes too. Being a math major, she could use that someday to be a researcher in the area of speech-language pathology.

I feel as if I was ready to leave the field, or really not liking it, around year seven or eight. I had a year where I happened to be on the non-public staff, and the day before school started, they switched me to the public staff. I did not have a lot of control over what school I was going to, and what school hours I would work. I thought, Is it worth it? Maybe it's the seven year itch or something. That also would be my advice to people, to try to get through that, and then see where you're at.

RW: Do you have any regrets, and would you do it all again?

SLP: Yeah, I would do it again. It worked out for me.

I Would Not Do It Again

RW: So what drew you to the field of speech pathology?

SLP: So originally I didn't know what I wanted to do. I knew I wanted to maybe teach. When I was little I was always interested in teaching, because my mom was a teacher, and I've always known people in the education field. So I ended up talking to my family about it, and my mom worked with an SLP and an OT [occupational therapist] when she was a teacher. She was like, "Hey, maybe you would be interested in this." I've always had a love of languages and I'm kind of a grammar nerd. I definitely kind of fell into it in that way. It wasn't like an authentic passion of mine, but I kind of grew to love it, and I ended up majoring in it in school. That's the short answer.

Also my dad had a traumatic brain injury, and he had two strokes. Years before I was born, he got into a bad car accident and sustained a TBI [traumatic brain injury]. And then he had a stroke because of that, he had a brain bleed. He later ended up having open heart surgery, and he then had another stroke because of some complications. He has had a long medical history, and as a result of that he had some language deficits and reading difficulties, as would be expected. I grew up kind of having to take charge if we went places, either to help my dad communicate with other people or communicate for him in a way, because he has difficulty advocating for himself or just getting people to understand what he's talking about. That's a personal reason that I ended up choosing it as well.

RW: So in the field so far, what's been frustrating?

SLP: I wish that I had known just how extroverted I needed to be. It's been very, very challenging for me because I didn't realize this, but I am more of an introvert than I thought I was. I'm actually doing teletherapy right now. I just finished my day, and I had sessions back to back. You're constantly having to be energetic in front of students. If I'm having a low energy day, I don't want them to feel that. I feel like I'm putting on a performance so to speak at work every day. So that's definitely one personal challenge.

I guess a professional challenge has just been that I feel a lack of respect from administrators and teachers. I just feel like no one really knows exactly what I do, or even if they do, there's just a lot of demands placed on you that sometimes are inappropriate. I'll just give you an example. Last school year. I was working for a public school. For a little over a year I worked for them, and it was the worst experience. I'll say hands down it's actually the reason why I ended up working in teletherapy right now.

RW: What was happening?

SLP: A few things happened. Last year I was an itinerant pre-K community person. Basically my job was traveling to different daycares and Head Starts and providing the services at their centers, and my caseload would change constantly. It was in a range of anywhere from no less than 35 students to upwards of 45 or 50, and I was case managing 80% of my cases.

RW: That's a lot.

SLP: Yeah, it was a lot. All of the students weren't actually at the center. We also had walk-in students. They would come to us. I agreed to do half community and half walk-in students. I was supposed to be 100% pre-K, but they used me to do other walk-in students too, because they had no one else to do it. It was just a mess. There was a huge lack of space. I didn't have an actual treatment space. I was eventually assigned a conference room with huge adult furniture, which was totally inappropriate for the kids. The kids would get up and run around the room, and I even got kicked out of the conference room multiple times by my own manager.

It was just this whole lack of respect thing. I was complaining, which in hindsight I probably shouldn't have been doing as much as I was, but I was just so frustrated with how things were being managed that I would talk about it to my coworkers. I guess my manager found out about that, and she ended up calling me into her office to discuss it. Of course I try to be professional, so I say, "I apologize, and I just feel frustrated with how things are being handled right now, and I don't feel like I'm being treated like a professional." I wasn't getting email responses from her either when we had community issues. There were a lot of things going on that year that were very frustrating, and she ended up threatening my evaluation because she was like, "Oh technically, you're a first year SLP, so you should be careful with how you're conducting yourself."

RW: Now, can I just say something supportive of you?

SLP: Of course.

RW: She was disrespectful to you. You're an adult, you're a professional. And she was doing that because you were young and you were new.

SLP: I think so too. I agree, well thank you for that.

RW: Really awful.

SLP: It was an awful situation and I'm glad that I moved on to something else. To be treated like you're less than, or you're not a professional and you don't know what you're doing, it's just very discouraging.

RW: What keeps you going anyway?.

SLP: I would say when the kids have their moments of just being funny, just being kids, their silly moments. That's definitely my number one thing. If the kids were not fun to deal with, I would just be like, I don't know what I'm doing here. I'll be honest, I think I'm at a point where there's not really anything which I might not be able to find in a different job or different career. I don't like the fact that I'm in this situation where I just feel like I want to leave. I'm currently looking at some other options, something that offers me something that fits me, my personality, a little bit better. I feel like I could possibly transition to something else that is more rewarding and more worth it for me to put my time and energy and effort into, because I would say most days are very draining for me, unfortunately.

I think more people in the general public, and especially regular ed teachers, special ed teachers, principals, admin, need to receive more education about speech pathology. I know that some school districts might have the SLPs talk about what it is that we do, what areas we can help with, and what goals we can work on. I feel like some people ask you to do things that I don't really know if I should be working on.

Also, we can educate about what we need. We need a quiet location, at least some sort of stable location, so the students know, okay, I'm going to the speech room now, and this is what I'm gonna be doing. I find that a lot of people complain about the fact that they don't have a stable or quiet space to work. I feel like it comes down to this lack of respect. It's like they don't think that our job is worthy enough of having our own classroom or space to work. I feel like that's a big thing.

RW: Do you have a story to share?

SLP: We had these bi-weekly meetings, and they were boring. The most useless, terrible, redundant meetings I've ever been to in my life. They were micromanaging our schedules, actually a huge part of life there was just their micromanaging in an aggressive way. At the last meeting that I was in with them before I ended up resigning, I was trying to say something about it. One of the higher ups was insinuating that what I had to say was not of value, and she's like, "We're just gonna move on." I think I said something like, "Well, can I please finish my point?" I finished my point, and I stood up and left after I finished talking, because I was so down. It was so rude and unnecessary.

RW: What advice would you give to someone entering the field?

SLP: My advice to them would be to really think about what you value as a person, and what kind of personality you have, and what kind of personality the field requires for you to have. I would say this: Before a person considers spending six plus years in school, I would definitely say to think about your personality. Also shadow SLPs before jumping in, because I wish I had done way, way more shadowing than I did beyond just the required observation hours. I feel like I didn't really get a good enough idea before starting. If I could go back, I definitely would have been like, All right, I'm gonna run away from here.

RW: Any regrets? And would you do it all again?

SLP: I do regret not looking into it more. I don't think I really even realized the education requirements. I didn't realize I even needed a master's, I'll be honest, until my orientation. I wish I had known that and I wish that I shadowed more to make it a more informed decision. I also think that familial pressure was hanging over my head, so I was just kind of going with it. I wish I had the strength at the time to say, "Okay, this isn't working out for me," because I think you know yourself better than anyone else. Then ask, "What can I do now, what can I do instead, using the skills in the areas that I'm interested in?" No, being honest, I would not do it again.

You Always Question Yourself

RW: Why did you become a speech therapist?

SLP: I started off going into special education because my cousin was doing that and it sounded like something I would enjoy. I helped her out a little bit, and then I did an internship in special education and realized I did not want to work with a full classroom. But I thought I would like to work with just a few kids at a time. When I went to college they had a careers book and I went through it, and it mentioned speech therapy. I thought, That sounds really interesting, so I'll go that route.

RW: What would you have become If you didn't become a speech therapist?

SLP: If I didn't become a speech therapist, I would really have enjoyed something in the fitness field. I really love that. Maybe cardiac rehab or even some kind of sports medicine.

RW: What frustrates you about our field?

SLP: Where to start? I have a few things. Working in the schools, the caseloads are so high that it's really difficult to make progress, and it's hard to get things done. You have 80 kids on a full-time caseload, and then you have to do the paperwork, the evaluations, IEPs [Individualized Education Plans], and meet all the timelines. You also work with students on intervention, which is not even counted in that caseload. I think it's sort of an impossible task, and it's not fair to the students. The other thing that frustrates me is the field is so broad, that if you're working in the schools, you have to work with kids with any disability, whether it's stuttering, a language issue, autism, whatever. And I don't think that anyone can be perfect at everything. It's really hard and it makes you doubt yourself sometimes.

RW: I've heard other people say they feel that the field is so broad that it's overwhelming.

SLP: You don't feel that sense of success, because you just can't get great at it. I think working in another setting where you specialize in a couple of different areas might be better for the students and the therapist.

RW: I think a lot of us have imposter syndrome. We know more than we think we do, but we never feel like we really know what we're doing.

SLP: I've had that for 35 years.

RW: What keeps you going anyway, even though it's frustrating. Why do you keep doing it?

SLP: It's too hard to change at this point to go into something else, so I'm kind of locked in, and with the State Teachers Retirement System, you're kind of locked into that. I do love working with the kids, just spending time with them seeing a little progress that you experience, mostly with articulation.

RW: Is there anything else that you find rewarding?

SLP: Spending time with the students and getting to know them. Making connections and giving them time, especially after everything with COVID and being off. I think just being there for them, giving them a place to feel safe and to talk. I think that's the number one most rewarding thing.

RW: What needs to change in our field to make it more workable?

SLP: Number one, lower the caseload size, it's ridiculous and impossible. Don't make us do these long workload calculators to figure out caseloads. It makes it really hard and just adds to the stress. I would say just a maximum caseload, weighted [based on type of disability] size, would be 60. I mean, I think it would still be high, but it would be doable. Actually 35, 40 would be ideal.

RW: What advice would you give to someone starting out in our field?

SLP: I have student teachers. And one piece of advice I always tell them is: I know it's scary and they feel insecure about starting, but you just have to jump in and do it, and then you keep tweaking it and changing it as you go. You're never going to be perfect at it. It's a learning process through the whole career. So just be patient and don't expect too much of yourself. You want to learn, but you shouldn't be too hard on yourself, because they make it very difficult with the caseload numbers.

RW: Any regrets, and would you do it all again?

SLP: I don't know. If I had it to do over, I might change fields, but I don't know. At one point, I kind of wished that I tried working in a different school district, but at this age I'm thinking it probably wouldn't have made a difference. I do enjoy working with the students that grow up in poverty and struggle a lot. I really enjoy that. I love working with the Latino population. Maybe I'd just do a different area of the field. I do feel like I'm good at some things with this job, but I still question all the time and worry that I'm not giving enough. You know, you always question yourself.

It's Not Age, It's Expertise

RW: Why did you become an SLP? What drew you to the field?

SLP: I got my bachelor's degree in Montessori education, early childhood three to six. I was a preschool and kindergarten teacher for six years. I was teaching and I was bored, and I thought If I'm bored, my students are bored. This is not good. I need to look around. At the time, my state was talking about requiring teachers to get their master's degree. I thought, Well, if I'm gonna have to go back to grad school, I don't really want to do more education. I'm already bored.

I happened to have two or three students in my class who received speech therapy, and I remember asking the speech therapist about one particular kid, "Hey, what are you working on? Is there anything I can do to help you in the classroom?" I mean, the questions that I asked are a speech therapist's dream, I know that now. She completely shut the door on me. She said, "Oh no. He's fine." I think she might have handed me a piece of paper and said "Here, send this home for his homework." I mean, she was not interested in collaborating with me or getting my help.

Because she did that, it made me do my own research. The more I researched it, the more I thought, I want to do this for a living. I was a newlywed at the time and talked to my new husband about quitting my job, and going back to school full time. We were in a position where I could do that. So, I did, and graduated. I think I had just turned 30 when I got my speech pathology degree. I was significantly older than my classmates. That's what happened, and I love it.

RW: I know you said you love it, but are there aspects of the field that frustrate you?

SLP: Well, I love my school, I love my caseload, I love my staff, but I hate that the district makes us carry the state maximum. You know we're carrying 80 kids. I was actually just talking to an intern about this today.

My district-specific frustration is the inherent systematic racism of working in an inner city school, where they make us carry these high caseloads. If we went anywhere in a middle class district, which is going to be traditionally more white, the caseloads are lower. They have the ability to give kids more intensive therapy in the suburbs, but not in the inner city, and it frustrates me. It really does frustrate me. it's inherent in the system. Say it however you want to say it, but that's what this is. They have got to get us lower caseloads because we'll be more effective. I know it's about money.

Of course the general field frustration is everything else we have to do besides actually working directly with the kids. But that's part of it, you just kind of have to figure out your own style, and your own way not to drown in the paperwork and the documentation and the Medicaid billing or the insurance billing. It's just part of the job. It's the least fun part of the job.

RW: What about our field in particular keeps you going?

SLP: Well, the kids. I've been at my school for nine years and I know the caseload really well. First and foremost, I just love working with the kids. Pediatrics is absolutely my area. I also love the staff, the Special Ed staff that I work with. I think we're a really great team. When I'm feeling down or thinking about how many kids I have to see that day, just a smile from my school psychologist, or kind word from the intervention specialist is always very nice to get. Honestly, it's the thing that's kept me going. This year it's a little bit different because I have had an intern with me since January for the second semester, and had the ability to pass on what I know, and train and teach somebody who's then gonna go out and do it too. I tell them I learn just as much from them. They're fresh out of school and can teach me things, and I'm always looking for new methods and new research and new materials. So it's the people. It's a people oriented field and that really is what keeps me going.

RW: What else do you find especially rewarding?

SLP: Well, being able to exit a kid who's reached their goals and gotten to where they can do things independently. It's always bittersweet whenever I exit a kid, they take it kind of as a rejection sometimes, and say, "But I like seeing you!" So we talk about how sad I am not to get to work with them, but how proud I am that they can do it all by themselves. They used to need my help and now they don't need my help, they can do it all by themselves and that gives them a sense of pride. I love those moments, and I love being able to say to the kids, "You can do it all by yourself now, you don't need me anymore." That's very satisfying.

RW: Do you have a favorite story?

SLP: It's a multitude of stories from the same student who's now in fifth grade. I've known him since he was in kindergarten, so for years I've been working with this guy, and he just always seemed to have just a really matter of fact way of putting things that made me want to laugh out loud, but I would wait till he left the room. He bumped his head one time while walking. He was trying to walk out the door backwards, which did not work out well for him. I said, "Are you okay?" And he said, "Yeah, I got a big head." So just my favorite moments are these funny little things that just pop out of kids. Then one time I had a materials box that looked kind of like a takeout box, it was red, and he pointed to it and said, "You got chicken in there?" I guess there used to be a TV show about kids that said the darndest things. I feel like we live that.

RW: You've got an intern this semester. What advice do you give them or for someone starting out in the field?

SLP: I am proud to say that my current intern has just gotten a job with my district, and she's my fourth intern to get hired by the district. There's a couple of things that I always make sure that I tell them. I always remind them as they're getting ready to graduate and they're looking for jobs, or they just got a job, that they have to remember that they're the expert in the room. So many times you are the only person there from our profession. Especially in the schools, you're the only SLP there and you're certainly the only SLP on a team. And you may only be 23 years old walking into an IEP [individualized education plan] meeting, or any kind of meeting about a kid, or meeting with a particularly challenging parent. You have to remember that you are the one who knows the field. So I always encourage them to remember it's not their age, it's their expertise. Because they're scared. I remember, we were all scared walking into that first meeting.

Then I also remind them that just because they are the island in the school, in one sense, they're also not alone in that there's an entire system. Wherever you work, there's some kind of system of support, whether it's in a clinic, a hospital, or a school district. You're given a supervisor for a reason. You're not supposed to just stay out there and drown. They have to remember that we all ask each other questions. I've been in speech for 25 years and I'm still reaching out to people and saying, "How do I treat this?" They always need to make sure that they're looking out for themselves in both of those ways.

RW: What change would you like to see in the field at large?

SLP: The field is getting so diverse. I know we have things like professional development that we have to keep up on, and ASHA is a great resource for keeping your training up and learning new skills. But I think the field is so diverse that I wish there was a way to find a particular path to go in. I had to do a stint in the nursing home, but I was miserable. I don't know if there's a way to whittle it down. I understand why they want students to get a look at how wide the field is, but I wish there was a way to pair down the training so that you could learn the skills that you really need.

RW: Would you do it all again?

SLP: I probably would have gone straight into the communication field. But then I might have deprived myself of some good behavior management skills. Although I didn't like teaching, I felt like I was a good teacher. I always had good control over my kids, so they learned what they needed to do. So as soon as I say I would just skip the teaching part, I think I would have deprived myself of some basic skills working with kids, because behavior management is a big thing that we have to figure out. And even for two, three, or four kids, it's still herding cats.

RW: Any regrets about becoming a speech therapist?

SLP: None here, I can honestly say zero percent. Zero. I love it. And like I said, I think it's because I started out on the "wrong path." I'll use those words in quotes. I started out in a field that I decided I wasn't happy about, and man when I landed here I have never looked back. I love it. It's so flexible, the field is so flexible. You can work with any age, any disability, any kind of environment.

Tania On *General Hospital*

RW: So what made you interested originally in speech pathology?

SLP: I have kind of a weird story. I knew I wanted to go into a healthcare field. My dad had spina bifida, and was in a wheelchair, so I was around disabled people. I wanted to be a physical therapist but knew I probably couldn't hack the science part of everything. At the time, *General Hospital* was a big soap opera that I watched. On *General Hospital*, there was Tony, who was the doctor, and Tania was his wife who was a speech therapist. They never showed what she did, but it sparked my interest to start looking into it, and that's what led me to speech therapy. So I knew at a pretty early age that I wanted to become a speech therapist and picked my undergrad college accordingly. The irony of the whole thing is, I worked with a girl when I first moved here who had the same story, that she got into speech therapy because of *General Hospital* too!

RW: What would you have become if you had not been a speech therapist?

SLP: Because I knew it at such an early age, I didn't really have any other strong likes. I mean, I love cooking. I always thought being a caterer or something would be fun. But I don't know if I could do that. I always thought about being a wedding planner because I like to be very organized. But then to deal with the Bridezillas, I didn't know if I could do that, either. So those are the things that sparked my interest, but I think because I knew for such a long time that I wanted to be a speech therapist I never thought seriously about anything else.

RW: Are you still working? What area are you in?

SLP: I have always worked primarily in outpatient adult rehab. I work in an outpatient clinic and I see adults with strokes, head injury, concussion, and voice disorders. I started my career here and I work for the same company that I have ever since I started. Early on in my career, there was a point where I worked at a major hospital that had acute care, rehab, outpatient and a SNF [skilled nursing facility]. At one point, I was a float therapist so I would float to all of those areas depending on the need. I've dabbled in all of those areas, but my first and foremost love is adult rehab.

RW: What frustrates you about our field?

SLP: Well, this is the biggest thing that I talk about, and all my friends that have been in this field as long as I have kind of agree. We went into this field because it was a helping profession and we wanted to help people. The company that I worked for, when I first started, that was their mantra: patient care, patient care, whatever you needed to do to provide the good patient care. Then in 2018 our company went into a joint venture. So I went from a not-for-profit to a for-profit, and the mentality changed. Right now it's very productivity driven. I understand it's a business, but we kind of have lost that it's all about the patient, and we've morphed it into whatever we can do to make money.

Productivity standards-it's getting to the point where it's unsustainable, and that's what I'm trying to get my employer to understand. They've reduced me to 45 minute sessions, except for evaluations for which I get an hour. The expectation is that I'm scheduled with 10 patients in an eight hour day. The thought process is that there'll be cancellations, so you'll have paperwork time, but that doesn't happen. They don't understand that our documentation is different from physical therapists and occupational therapists who can document point-of-service. I choose not to, because I think it goes against our standard of what we're trying to work on, which is communication and eye contact and pragmatics, and my head in a computer is not how I want to treat patients. So I bring a lot of my paperwork home. I do one to three hours of paperwork each night, and I get burned out. I keep telling them that. I have 32 years in the same company, so my seniority and my PTO [paid time off] is so high that I can't really afford to leave. I can't find something that's gonna match my salary or compensate for that PTO. So I'm just trying to stick it out.

I'm uber frustrated right now. Our company has multiple clinics throughout the city. The other clinic that's closest to me has a therapist who went out on maternity leave, and they chose not to cover her maternity leave. Those patients are being transferred to me. I was on medical leave too, and came back with an incredibly full schedule with about four to five evals a day. There comes a point that there's no more treatment spots. Right now I have no openings on my schedule until months from now. It's very, very difficult for me to evaluate a patient who's just had a stroke and tell them, "I'm sorry, I can't see you for months." So I book them over my lunch hour.

I've talked to my supervisor about it, and I've talked to the person above her, and they simply either don't care or don't know what to do. The comment that my manager gave me is, "Yeah, when I saw your schedule when you came back from medical leave, it even made me anxious." I'm thinking, Well then why didn't you do something about it? My biggest frustration is that I've had two managers who were physical therapists tell me that I needed to learn how to document better. And there's nothing that frustrates me more, because when I was a manager, I never told another discipline how to do their job. And I've told both of them, "Please don't tell me how to do my job."

It's like, hey, follow me for a day, I go back to back to back to back. I had a patient yell at me because I chose to go to the bathroom. I was about five minutes late going to get her, and she got pissed at me. And I'm just like, I don't know what I'm supposed to tell you. She said, "Well, they should build that into your schedule." But the best part was that she was a nurse, so she should have understood! Another frustration is there's some insurance plans that are very restrictive here, because individuals who are on straight Medicaid who are over the age of 21 do not have speech benefits. So, if you're 30, on Medicaid, and have a stroke, and you can't talk, you don't get services.

RW: What do you find rewarding?

SLP: My patients. That's what keeps you going.The success that you see or the changes that you see. The best are the ones that after you discharge them, they come back and tell you how they're doing. That's why I accommodate my patients, especially the ones who are grateful for that. But then I also have to pay my mortgage and I have to buy food for my kids, so those things keep me going too.

RW: Do you have any favorite stories?

SLP: There was a patient that was involved in a car accident, and his car blew up in flames. He was so disfigured, so badly burned. He eventually came to our rehab, and then to outpatient, and he became my patient. He had a lot of facial burns so we were working on facial stretching and trying to be able to open his mouth, and his goal was to eat a double cheeseburger from Jack in the Box. At one point, a gentleman that had witnessed the accident came to our session because he wanted to meet my patient. They were talking as I'm stretching the patient's mouth. This witness was apologizing because he couldn't get to the car in time to try to get the patient out. My patient said, "That's okay. It's okay, it's okay. I'm fine. You know, I'll be fine. I'll be fine." Oh my God, he was so accepting of what happened to him. He never made you feel like he was mad or irritated.

And then one day we were walking through the clinic, and there was a gentleman there who was in a power wheelchair, and he used an electrolarynx because he had a gunshot wound to the neck, so he couldn't use his voice. My patient, who's completely disfigured top to bottom, looks at me and says, "Oh my God. Thank God I'm not him."

RW: Whoa, that is incredible. Really inspiring! Switching gears completely, what do you think needs to change to make therapy more doable?

SLP: I think the big, big thing that needs to change is how we get reimbursed by insurance, because the fact is that they keep reimbursing us less and less every year. So in order to make it profitable, you have to see more patients. That's why I had to go to 45 minute sessions, so that I could get more patients in a day, so I could bill more. It's just going to keep getting worse and worse. I don't know that much about school systems, because I never worked there. But I feel in a way it's getting like that there too, because they hire the SLPAs to do all the treatment, and the therapist is the one who's writing the IEPs [Individualized Education Plans]. So they don't even know these kids, and they're writing all these IEPs. It's that whole theory of more work and less people.

RW: What advice would you give to someone starting out in our field?

SLP: I guess to be more open-minded. Our newer grads say that, "Oh, I don't want to do that, I don't want to do voice therapy." Or, "I'll see cancer patients, but only the ones that have cognitive problems and not the swallowing ones." Like when did we become able to dictate what diagnoses we see? We're finding new grads just don't do well in our environment right now. I think that's because it's so demanding from a billing productivity standpoint, but also because of the expectation of what you have to get done in a shorter amount of time. We hired a couple of new grads at a different clinic, and they just couldn't handle the paperwork and wanted two hours for an eval. And I'm thinking, honey, that's not the real world, I'm sorry.

Also, I'd say to new grads, you have to bring the patient in, because often what's written on the script is not what they wind up needing treatment for, or it's not a hundred percent accurate. I had one mother call me a while back. Her daughter had been shot in the face. When you read it on paper, she shouldn't have been able to talk or swallow. She was still fed via a PEG tube, and they wanted to get the PEG out, but no speech therapist would see her. I sent her for a swallow study, which was a hundred percent normal. I literally saw her twice and that was it. I'm like, so you guys refused to see her based on her diagnosis or the complex history that you read on the paper. And all it took was referring her for a swallow study. It's so frustrating that her mother had to spend all that time calling around trying to find somebody.

RW: Do you have any regrets?

SLP: It's not really a regret. I would just do it differently. When I came out of high school, I was very timid, introverted, and very shy. The school I chose to go to as an undergrad was a small women's Catholic college. I felt like I wanted that smallness. What I didn't realize is that it would limit my experience. Because we were so small, for clinicals and so forth we didn't have a lot of options. Plus it was a very educationally based program, so it was all geared towards therapists who would be working in the schools. Had I known more about that program as an undergrad, I probably would have done my undergrad somewhere else, but you can't change the past, and there's a reason for everything that happens.

RW: Would you do it again?

SLP: I probably would do it again. My daughter said, "Yeah, you'd do it again but you'd want a different outcome." But the thing is, everything that I would want to change to have a different outcome is way out of my control, right?

Paperwork and Pants

RW: What brought you to the field?

SLP: That's such an interesting question. I started as a theater major, and I took a voice and articulation class. My professor really appreciated my affinity for the topic. He said, "You know, you might think about being a speech therapist." But I didn't know anything about the topic. I didn't know it even existed as a career. I changed majors as a junior, and just in general fell in love with the field. There are so many options that you can choose, you can work with adults, you can work with children. I just thought it looked like a good career, but otherwise I would have been an actress.

RW: How many years of experience have you had in the field?

SLP: I would say 30. I had a 10-year gap there for a while. I started in the field, and practiced for a few years, and I could not deal with the emotional baggage that it came with. I just cried so many tears in my office. I was so young and I just thought I cannot look at a career doing this all the time. This is too much for me. So I did about a 10 year sabbatical. But then it called me back, because in the end I really was dedicated to the field of speech pathology.

RW: What frustrated you about the field?

SLP: Well, without a question, my biggest frustration is the ever growing paperwork. It was so frustrating and so monotonous. I thought, Why am I doing this? When I first started in speech, even in the schools, I could get a kid into speech with checklists. One from the parents, maybe a couple from different teachers. It was just no big deal to get a kid in. I understand the need for the process, I do appreciate and value the whole tier of interventions. But the amount of paperwork had absolutely destroyed any fun, any joy in my last couple of years. It was so painful that I'm still recovering.

RW: How did you keep going?

SLP: I hung in there in part because at some point you're so invested, you can't get out, and also because of the kids.

RW: So what you found rewarding was…?

SLP: Progress. I really did like working with the kids. I don't know that I was the funnest speech therapist. I didn't play a lot of games. But we dug into things that they needed. I am kind of relentless in some ways and so I gave them as much time as I could. We saw progress, and that made me happy. I even had kids tell me, "If it weren't for you, I would not have passed those tests." Brain development, child development, therapy techniques, we know a lot, and I don't think most people fully appreciate the depth of our knowledge.

 RW: Do you have any favorite stories?

SLP: Yes.This kid was so beautiful. He was in a preschool class of students with multiple disabilities and he was identified as autistic. He was mainly nonverbal. He loved coming to school, and he loved speech. I had taken a small group into my office, and it had been a great class. This child was just so happy, and all of us were happy. I was praising this group and telling them how much I love teaching them. He held his arms out to me, and he looked me bashfully in the eyes and he said, "Come here, Fatty girl." I was so excited because he had initiated this interaction! It was so appropriate, it was so relational. It was so perfect! And then I realized he called me fat!

There was another kid, too. This little guy was a preschooler, and he was an articulation [sound issue] kid. And there had been a couple snow days, so we had been interrupted for like three weeks. When we started our therapy session again, I said to him, "Do you remember what we're learning right now?" He said, "Well, I am learning to be a gentleman." I said, "You are. Huh. Well, what does a gentlemen do?" He said, "Well, I get beers for my mom."

RW: Those are great stories! What advice would you give to someone starting out in our field?

SLP: The big piece of advice is keep your eye on the ball, which is that child's, or that client's, communication skills.

RW: Any regrets, and would you do it again?

SLP: Oh, I absolutely would, but I would definitely not be a school based SLP. I would have to do something else because the amount of paperwork is directly proportional to the size of my pants.

Go Ahead, Just Pick Me a Major

RW: What drew you to the field of speech language, pathology?

SLP: I actually started out in college as a business major, and I kind of ran through that whole department, trying to find a niche that worked for me. It wasn't a good fit. My roommate at the time said, "Let me go get the big book of majors." I thought, Sure, why not? It's kind of that crazy moment where anything could happen. She said, "Well, what do you like?" I said, "Well, I like language but I don't want to be a writer, and I love education, but I don't want to be a teacher. I'm not someone who could be up in front of 25 kids. I love the medical field, but I don't want to be a doctor or a nurse, because science is not necessarily my thing. Just go ahead, pick me a major!" It was one of those three in the morning things. She starts reading about speech pathology. It's talking about education classes, there are language classes, and there's medical and there's psychology. So I registered for a summer intro class. I just fell in love with it. I was just fascinated, and immediately felt like, yeah, this is it.

RW: As much as we love our field, there are some frustrations. What have you found frustrating?

SLP: I was in the middle of my CF [clinical fellowship] in the skilled nursing facility. I hated every second of it, because of all the things they don't tell you about in school that you have to learn. I was expected to have 90% productivity. I thought, I'm a hard worker, I'm an efficient person, I can do this, right? I was never taught how to build a caseload. So here I am not really having a caseload, not really having a supervisor that did anything. I didn't feel like I knew what to do. I had two buildings, and I had maybe two or three people at each building, which was not enough for a full-time job. In school, I remember learning you don't pick up people for therapy that should not be picked up. You pick up the people that are appropriate, so it's ethical; you're gonna help these people and you're gonna make it better. So they bring me these people that clearly were not appropriate. They said, "Oh well, that's what you do." And I'm like, "No, I'm not, I'm not supposed to do that," right? You know, bright-eyed therapist. So, I'm not making money to pay my bills. I don't know what I'm going to do. I hate the work I'm doing because I already felt like just a warm body. I was so frustrated, and ready to leave.

Now, when I did my supervision as a student, my supervisor was amazing. She was wonderful, and I thought, Boy, I'm gonna have one just like that. I realized it just isn't like that after graduation. I'd have patients that I wanted to work with, so I'm thinking, Okay, what's practical? What can we do? What's gonna be really great therapy? "Oh, you can't do really great therapy because you can't bill to work with another therapist at the same time as you, because then we can't make as much money for that. So you just go about working with this comatose patient for an hour. Make sure you elevate her diet so that everybody's happy, whether it's appropriate or not."

I wasn't helping. I felt like a fraud. I felt terrible and I was trying to figure out how to make this work so that I could support myself and my field, meet this unrealistic percentage, but do what I'm actually supposed to be doing and help somebody. I just felt like it was nothing like what I thought it was going to be.

I remember as a student, I was only allowed to work with Medicare Part A people. Guess what? Those are the best of the best, the people that have a strong potential to improve. They've maybe just had their stroke or maybe they've just come off of an accident, and then they're ready to go and are a lot more motivated. Well, you know what? When I got to the nursing homes, it was all the people that have been there for 20 years. There is a running joke in my house. I had a lady that had dementia for many, many years. I went to my supervisor at the time, who I really liked, he happened to be a PTA [Physical Therapy Assistant]. I said, "I just don't feel like I'm making a difference for anybody," and I was so upset. He said "No, you know what? When you started working with that lady five weeks ago, all she could do was say 'blah blah blah,' but now she can go 'BLAH BLAH BLAH,'" and I laughed. I know that sounds terrible, but he was trying to make me feel better.

But that was less than nine months in, and I already was wondering, What am I doing? Once I finished my CF I felt as if I had a little more freedom to move. I found a private clinic associated with a hospital. We did private outpatient visits with patients from birth to 100 plus. We also did the contract for the hospital. You had the Modifieds [radiographic swallow tests], and you had the acute inpatient, and a lot of it was the evals and then the quick patient turnover, but I loved it. I never knew what my day was going to be, and I thought, This is amazing. This is a great job.

But I was salaried, and I took a huge pay cut. So then I had to work four to five PRN [called in when needed] jobs, an additional three to four hours a night or even more sometimes, to make up. So here I am loving my job, and I'm at least making a guaranteed number. I remember I was overloaded with stress and my now-husband said, "You've got to not take on more than one PRN job at a time." I just kept taking more, though, because the money kept coming in and I was paying off debts, but I was going crazy. You know what I mean?

RW: I do!

SLP: So this was private practice. I loved my work, I loved so many things about it, but then I had to work all these extra hours just to make it financially worth it for me. After my husband and I got married, we moved into a state that needed therapists in the schools. I found a school right near where we lived, it was an elementary school. I loved that school, but I had 80 plus kids on my caseload. It was still so much. We had a union rep who all of us therapists told, "Hey, we need to talk to you, because this is what's coming our way, and we're still on this teacher pay scale." I think so many of us speech people are just so driven. We're gonna get this done, this is what we do. I think as a rule we're very organized people and we manage, and we say, "We're gonna do this job well," but it doesn't mean that we're not suffering as a result of it.

Later I took a different job at a private practice. I loved it, but I feel like when you're the speech person the rules change depending on whoever decides to set them, and you're kind of just stuck with it. They started telling me we have another speech friend, and she's recommending that you do these therapies. I said, "Why don't you hire HER?" They were talking about oral motor skills, but what I had been reading said that they do not show carry over of skills into speech production. This clinic was pediatric, it was all kiddos. I said, "You know, a lot of our kids only get 10 covered therapy visits a year, right? I want to maximize what I'm doing with them. So, this is my plan, and this is why I'm gonna do it." They said, "Well, why don't you take a session or two to do what we're asking, and then tell them why it doesn't work?" I said, "I'm not gonna do that. That is wasting their time and I'm not okay with that. That is not in their best interest and if I know better, I'm gonna do better." They were physical therapists, so I said, "I don't tell you how to do your practice."

RW: A lot of frustrations.

SLP: So a lot of frustration, I just want to do what I do, and I feel like no one really wants to let me and pay me a fair wage. We had twins back in December of 2010. That was my out with that clinic. Then at some point I heard about teletherapy. That's where I'm at now. This job is full-time. It is salaried. I don't want to get paid by the kid because I know that many are no-shows.

To be honest, I don't really love this job, either. I've thought so many times about leaving the field, but I feel trapped because this is all I'm trained to do. I could go and maybe work at a desk somewhere, maybe work at a grocery store, sell flowers, or do something like that, and earn ten dollars an hour. For my family that's not okay. I just want to work, but I don't want to feel miserable at work.

My favorite thing ever was working with the two and three year olds, the ones that were the delayed talkers. You get that kid that has behaviors that are coming out of their not being able to communicate, but then one day, it clicks for them. Like, if I just use my words or something else to get my point across, I can get that toy that I want. It clicks, and that is going to get that ball rolling. It just takes off from there, and that's like my "Aha!" moment, and I live for that!

RW: Would you do it all again?

SLP: You know, that's hard. I love it and I'm fascinated by it. I think it's valuable, I think it's worthwhile, and I've seen the outcome of it. I don't know what else I would go back and do. We just get it done, and they think because we get it done we can handle it. So they let us do it, or they even give us more, because they think we're fine. **But** I'm not fine. I just get it done.

RW: What drew you to being a speech therapist? What appealed to you about it or interested you?

SLP: I was floundering around in college and had no idea what I wanted to do until my third year. I took a communications class with the football coach's wife, who was a speech pathologist, and I connected with her. I really didn't know what I was getting into, but I knew enough to know that I would always have a job if I could get through grad school. That's kind of how I ended up doing it. There was no, "Oh, I'm in love with the field and this is what I want to do." It was just something that connected and I knew I could do it. It came fairly easily, I understood what I was studying pretty quickly and felt like it was a good fit.

RW: Can you think of anything else that you would have been?

SLP: I would have gone into the Peace Corps, that was essentially where I was headed. I was working on a social worker degree. My dad was like, "It's ridiculous, you won't make any money. How are you gonna support yourself? Everybody burns out in that field." So that's probably the direction I would have gone had I not had a little bit of guidance, looking back. Now, you know my interest really is in real estate and houses and that kind of stuff. I don't have any background or training but that is something of high interest to me now, that I wish I would have gotten into.

RW: Tell me about your experience in the field.

SLP: So, I am 33 years in, almost all of my experience has been pediatric: early intervention, school-based. I've owned and run a clinic for 10 years. I've been an independent contractor for most of the time. I've worked in the Alaskan bush for a good portion of that, and that's where I started my career. I worked for the school district there part time, then did independent contracting. I did a couple of stints traveling in Washington, and then ended up in New Mexico, where I've been doing more independent contracting, mostly to Indian reservation schools.

RW: Talk to me a little bit about the cultural differences in the clients that you work with and how you work within that.

SLP: Alaska was a really good place to start and I was placed in Anchorage originally. Alaska doesn't have a school that turns out speech pathologists, and especially not back 30 some years ago. So it was all high recruitment and I was put into one school. I had a hundred and thirty kids probably on my caseload as a CF [clinical fellow]. It's rough. However, the money was good coming right out of school. It was a good salary and it was an adventure, because I was young and ready.

I stuck with that job on a part-time basis for as long as I did, almost 20 years, because of the support that I had from the administration there. I was given the freedom to try out different settings, different kinds of jobs. I was able to go into administration eventually in Anchorage, with the support of a really strong supervision team. I think that is probably the only reason I'm still in this field, and have the dedication that I have to it. It's probably because of those foundational pieces. I had a lot of support early on and was given a lot of opportunity to screw up and still come out of it. The people that ran that program were themselves speech pathologists, so they had worked their way up into higher administration. Anchorage is a huge school district and so there was a lot of opportunity there for me to try.

Things were a lot different there. Culturally the school that I was in was a melting pot, and a huge native population would come in from the bush and be there from October until April, and then would leave.They'd miss school every year. But I learned a lot about the Native population, in particular, in Alaska, that really carried over to all of the jobs that I've had down here in New Mexico. Especially for us as speech pathologists, because we value oral communication so much and they don't. Trying to walk that fine line of yes, they want them to talk, but they only want to talk so much. Reading body language and all of that, that was a great learning experience.

RW: What frustrates you the most in the field?

SLP: I got a divorce and I needed to leave Alaska. Again, 20 years in, so I was well compensated in Alaska and my years of experience meant something to that district. But when I started looking, I was shocked by the number of big companies that have come in and taken over the field, and really don't value whether you have experience or not, they just want your license. There was no way really for me to go into a school district and make anything close to what I was making before. I was now responsible for the insurance of my family, and the amount of money that they were offering with benefits was not enough to sustain me and my kids. I was shocked by that. I just never would have guessed that would be the situation.

 I think it's really really difficult for us to move on to other positions. I wasn't interested at that point in administration. I had done it and knew that I probably did not want to work more hours again. I have a special needs kid and we were in the throes of that. So I would say the frustration right now is that it's kind of a dead-end job. There's not a lot of places to go if you want to make any decent money at this. It looks to me like independent contracting is the primary way to go, but we don't have benefits, and we don't have retirement. We only get paid if we can work. That was great until about three years ago when I got COVID, like the kind where I was in a coma and about died. I was down for about three weeks intubated and in a coma.

RW: Oh my God.

SLP: Yeah, it was a big deal. It was an eye-opener.

RW: How awful that you had to go through that. I'm so sorry.

SLP: I mean it was terrible, but luckily I had been paying for my own insurance, so I had insurance coverage. But no income of course came in for a good six months. I was coasting, and it really made me sort of assess my situation, and I am still. That's why I'm in Mexico. I am here trying to figure out how to live out the next 15 years, because I've probably got another good 15 years of work that I need to do to make enough to live on, and also live fairly comfortably.

I really can't do that in the states right now unless I'm willing to take on a big job. I'm going back next week, but my plan is to move here permanently in June. I think I can get insurance here, but even if I can't, my medical situation has improved tremendously and I can pay as I go. For instance, this morning, I went to the dentist and it cost $35 to get a full cleaning. I'm gonna need a mouth guard for TMJ and that's gonna cost me another $45. It's very inexpensive here and I live in an area that's full of expats.

So I should tell you too, that I ran a clinic for 10 years and I worked very closely with three of the state universities in New Mexico. Part of my practice was built on being at a trainee facility for therapists, whether they were doing their rotations, or they were in their CF, or whatever. I thought it was just tragic to listen to them telling me what they were making. You know, they had taken $200,000 or $250,000 loans to get through school. I knew they were going to come out and make $45 an hour with no benefits. It's really, really hard to consult and say, "Oh yeah, this is a great field right now." It might look okay to some of these new grads. That money sounds a whole lot better than minimum wage, right? I haven't found a lot of ability to grow, and I am also seeing the money go down. Money that I would have made 15 years ago, $50 an hour, that isn't even necessarily the norm anymore in a lot of places. I've seen people post things at $38 paid on a1099 [tax form] and I'm like, "How are you living?"

RW: That's not tenable.

SLP: It's not, it's hard, especially because this has been a field that I have been passionate about. When I opened my clinic, I always had a job, I've always had work. I may have had to be creative about what I did, but it was possible. I'm not sure it is possible anymore for some of these young guys coming out.

I am working. I do love the children and I love the people that I'm working with, and as long as I am contracting through my own contract, I make enough money to make it work. So that's what's keeping me going right now, but I have been very actively exploring other options. I think my other option is going to be teletherapy independent contracting for the foreseeable future. Again, I'll just kind of wait to see if something else sparks an interest. We have a broad base of skills, but it's also very difficult to make that transfer into other fields. When you do, you're starting over again. I just don't know that I want to start over at this age

RW: So what did you find most rewarding? I think you've kind of touched on that, but…

SLP: The relationship with the people that I work with, the children. I've loved working with families from the beginning. So early intervention has always been a very favorite thing of mine, especially out on the Indian reservations because it's such a big deal for them to allow you to be a part of their family. So when that happens it's really pretty cool.

RW: What else needs to change in our field?

SLP: There's no security. I don't have retirement other than what I've built for myself. For those of us in the educational field in particular, we are looking truly at a gig economy here, and I think that as professionals it really dumbs down our field in a lot of ways. When I've worked for big contracting companies, I've only done short stints for them. They didn't care, nor did the people who I was working with care, whether I knew how to do anything. I would be placed in a school, and luckily I knew schools. Nobody checked up on me. Nobody said, "Hey, we'd like to use you in this way, or we appreciate what you're doing." It was nothing. I was just a body that was thrown out to be there. That's how I felt.

RW: Completely switching gears here: Do you have a favorite story?

SLP: When I was in Alaska, and I had those 130 kids on that caseload, it was crazy. And 90% of that school was bilingual or monolingual in all different languages. There were different Asian communities, there were some Hispanic, but mostly they were from all over different parts of Asia. I had a child that was from Cambodia. It was during those weird school ground shooting things, so there was a big move of Laotian and Cambodian people to Alaska. I'm working this crazy case load, I'm barely functional. I'm in my CF here and I work with this child all year. Essentially, he was in a kindergarten classroom and he barely spoke English. I have no idea why he was on the caseload really to begin with, other than it was for language issues and somebody must have not been paying attention. So I work with him all year, and we bring the mom in for the IEP meeting, and she sits down. We start talking through an interpreter. I'm explaining what we're working on and I can tell, she's like, "What is this?" It turns out I worked for an entire year with a child who had the same name as another child that was of the same age and also in another kindergarten class. Stuff like that happens. It wasn't even possible to do that job, you know? At the time, because you're young, you think people are expecting you to do it. That was my story. I always tell that to my students so that they understand shit happens.

RW: What advice would you give to someone starting out in our field?

SLP: So they're already committed and in the field?

RW: We can look at that question in more than one way, however you want to look at it. Would you recommend someone going into this field right now?

SLP: I don't think so right now. And it makes me sad because a huge commitment of mine was paying it forward after I was treated so well in Alaska. It was important to me to be a good mentor and to really get people into the field and have them understand what to expect. But since leaving the clinic, which was about five years ago, I really struggled to find a whole lot of redeeming qualities in this. I think the right work situation would make a big difference, but it's been a struggle. I don't know that I would encourage anybody at this point to go into anything educational or medically related. But if they were already starting out my number one advice right now is to get rid of these corporate companies that have come in and are doing this. I feel like they are just destroying our field.

RW: They've bastardized it?

SLP: They have absolutely. Last night, there were like four different posts of people on Facebook saying they had an offer for $38 an hour on a 1099, and asking "What do you guys think about that?" And I saw somebody post, "Well, it depends on what area you're in. That might be competitive in Florida, but it might not be competitive here." And I was like, It's not competitive at all. **Thirty** percent off of the top of that goes to your taxes and self-employment. You're barely making minimum wage. You have to pay your own insurance. I think the first thing would just be truly coaching new students. I think it should be part of college because they are very, very stuck when they start taking these positions and there's just no place for them to go.

RW: Do you feel like part of the reason that we don't ask for what we deserve is because we're largely female? Do you think that's a piece of it?

SLP: Absolutely. I have that militant part of me which has really developed in the last 10 years. Oh my God, I can't believe this. People have all expected us to work these crazy caseloads, and they are paying us half price to do our paperwork time when it's not direct, and how is that acceptable in any other field? And it's not. What I'm hearing from people around our age is: I'm burnt out and done. If I could walk away from this field this second, I would be out.

That would be my advice to new students: set boundaries.I feel like a lot of them are a little bit more assertive than maybe I was back when I started out, because I just didn't know any better. I think that needs to be a huge part of what these people are trained for coming out of school.

RW: Would you do it all again? Any regrets?

SLP: I don't think I have regrets. I am feeling very stuck now, but this field supported me and my kids when I was really on my own with them. I always was able to have a job, and I was agile enough or flexible enough to figure out ways to make a living doing this. But it was hard. I mean, for the last five years that I had children at home, I had a nanny that covered those kids for two days a week while I was living down on an Indian reservation. That's how I made my living. I could bill a lot of money for that, but I had to have somebody else with my children in order to do that. I don't think there are a lot of people that are willing to do that kind of travel, and I don't necessarily recommend it, but it's what I had to do to survive.

RW: Yeah, as a single mom, you do whatever you have to do to put food on the table and have insurance.

SLP: I am glad that I have met incredible people and worked with just amazing people. I've been very, very lucky, but if I were going to college right now, this is not something that I would probably recommend to anybody until some of these things are cleaned up and addressed. I don't know when they're going to be addressed because I don't know how many people care right now. I think there needs to be really good representation at the younger end of things. If I had stayed in

Anchorage and finished my career there, I probably would have a very different perspective of this field. But because I had to make a move, boy, it changed it changed everything. And it really opened up my eyes to the fact that we are really very stuck in this field.

Move to Teletherapy

RW: So what brought you to speech therapy?

SLP: Last quarter of my freshman year, I took a phonetics course at college and I was hooked. I thought, Wow, this sounds really neat, and I changed my major from psychology to speech language pathology and audiology. When I was working in the schools, I thought if I wasn't an SLP, I'd like OT [occupational therapy]. Now I'm not quite so sure.

RW: You were telling me about how you really enjoy teletherapy.

SLP: I love it, it's one-on-one. There's no case management. You just have to do progress reports and annual reviews. You can do evaluations online as well. Right now, I contract with two companies who contract with virtual schools. They don't have their own related service staff, so they contract out. It's considered self-employment. Of course, you have to keep a third of your check aside for taxes. So now after retirement, this is what I'm doing. I can set my hours, my days.

RW: What frustrates you about our field?.

SLP: I was with public schools. I had a caseload of 80. It used to be 80 bodies, then they changed it to weighted, depending on the disability. Some students were weighted more heavily than others. If you had a weighted amount of 80, that was your limit. Quarterly progress reports, annual reviews, evaluations- it was terrible. It was a lot of paperwork, a lot of red tape, a lot of jumping through hoops. Some of the parents were telling me and other teachers what to do, or how to do it. Sometimes parents were not involved at all. That was very frustrating. Until our state changes that number of 80, nothing will change. Now, some school districts don't go by that, but here some of the public schools do, and it's just not manageable.

RW: What do you find rewarding?

SLP: It's one-on-one in teletherapy. I get to know the students. I get to know the families. I've had so many parents tell me how thankful they are, and how much progress they've seen in their students. While I could see that in the public schools, it was harder, or it took longer, because there were groups, and there were 80 kids to see in a week. I did like the collaboration in the schools. I could collaborate with the teachers or the OT or the intervention specialist, and here it is more isolated. Since I'm not a school staff person, I'm a contract person, it can be a little more difficult, but I reach out and almost always I get a favorable response.

RW: That's good to know. What would you like to see change in our field?

SLP: Oh, definitely a move to teletherapy. When all these school districts were literally thrown into it because of COVID, I was very frustrated because I knew there was a better way that it could be done. The staff could have been trained. I've been doing teletherapy for 10 years, so I knew there definitely was a better way to do it. Teachers were told to use Google Meet, they couldn't use anything else. And Google Meet did not have the features that Zoom had. So I knew it could have been handled a lot better. I do think everyone should be trained in teletherapy: medical, schools, nursing homes, whatever, in case the client can't come to the facility for speech, or in case something like this happens again. I think if everyone was trained, teletherapy would go a lot smoother.

There'd be better success than just saying, "Oh here: do teletherapy."

RW: It seems so much more efficient.

SLP: Yes and no. Some things are harder. I started with an AAC student three years ago. I'm thinking, How in the world do I do AAC [augmentative and alternative communication] using teletherapy? But that student has just blossomed. She has gone way beyond any expectations. Mom was such a great asset with modeling and being receptive to learning new things, showing her child where the icons were and things like that. So parents are definitely helpful. I think it can happen more with teletherapy than when you're in the schools.

RW: You have access to the parent and can train them? That's a real plus.

SLP: Absolutely, yes..

RW: Can you tell the story about the student that you ran into?

SLP: I've had a few of them and sometimes I hardly recognize them because they're adults. Then I'll hear them talk, and it's funny that I may not remember their names, but I remember what they worked on. So, in my head, I'm thinking Oh, you really carried over the articulation!

RW: Besides learning teletherapy, is there any other advice you have for people entering the field?

SLP: Learn sign language. I took a class in grad school, although it wasn't required. After I graduated and was working in the schools with the lower functioning kids, it was useful. I think sign language is essential, at least knowing basic sign language, because then you can pair the sign with the word or the picture.

RW: Would you do it all again?

SLP: Yes. You know, if you love what you do, it doesn't feel like work. It may have been frustrating in the schools, but I loved seeing the kids. I didn't like the paperwork and red tape and a lot of other things, but I like collaborating. I like working with the kids and I still do, and that's kind of what keeps me going.

Sign Me Up

SLP: I retired four years ago. Before that I worked in the schools. I was in charge of the preschool program, getting kids from birth to three into the preschool program and then doing all the preschool eligibility stuff. My specialty, other than my preschool kids, was teaching kids with reading disabilities to read.

I now work with two little kids. I know their families, and I work with them on reading. That's what I currently do. It was really hard for me to think that after I retired I wouldn't do anything. I just felt like something was missing, and it was weird because I didn't expect that. I think some of it is because you create such a bond with these kids and the families that when you don't have that, it feels like, okay, I gotta do something because I need that. I need that feeling again.

RW: It's the connection.

SLP: I mean I still have one family whose kids I saw 10 years ago and are now in high school, who contact me and talk to me and send me stuff about how the kids are doing. That's what it's about in my world.

RW: That's what you enjoy?

SLP: It's that bond thing and it's such a nice feeling. I don't know if when I first went into this field if that's what I expected, because I kind of happened upon speech therapy.

RW: So what brought you to the field? What else might you have become if not a speech pathologist?

SLP: Well, I first went to school to be an engineer. My father was an engineer, so I thought, I'll be an engineer, that sounds like something interesting. Then I met this girl that was going into the speech-language program. She was telling me about it, and I thought, Oh really, there's a job out there where I can just play games with kids? I mean, that's it. Sign me up for that job. I ended up taking the intro to communication disorders class, and I was just fascinated by it. I don't know what I would do differently if I wasn't in speech.

I was blessed in a way because I worked in my school job for a long time, but I never did school-based therapy. I was pretty much more like an admin making sure things ran smoothly and doing evaluations, and I love to do that. So I never had as much stress as a lot of the school-based speech therapists who actually did the treatment, because their caseloads were huge, and I thought God, I don't know if I could do that.

RW: It's exhausting. Did anything frustrate you about your career?

SLP: The things I think that frustrated me were when I saw certain things that needed to happen on the evaluation team, and changes that needed to be made, because I had done it for a long time. It was very difficult to get the administration to see that those changes needed to be made, and then make them, because every time I talked to them they would say, "Well, you guys are running so smoothly, you guys never need our help." And I said, "No, that's not really the issue. The issue is that we can make this better." Probably my most frustrating thing was parents who didn't call you back. You're on that birth to three timeline thing. Could you get those kids in by three?

RW: What kept you going through the years?

SLP: Probably more my outside interests and trying not to bring everything home from work. I love to do Pilates. I love to do yoga. So I had to continue to make sure that I built in time so that I could do that. Otherwise, I think that I would have felt that the job was just all-consuming. I needed an outside interest that I really liked. Hanging out with friends, going to places, but it honestly was probably more of the exercise component. If I start getting overwhelmed, and I go out and walk for a while, I'm fine. If I go do something that takes some effort, I do better.

I think that when you have such a large caseload in the schools, you just get so overwhelmed. I don't think you start to think about that self-care kind of stuff, and you don't do all the stuff that you need to do to manage your sanity

RW: What do you think needs to change in our field? What would you like to see change?

SLP: There seems to be such a disconnect between the people in the wide variety of areas that we can go into. I went into the reading part. Not very many speech therapists do reading. I think it would be really nice if ASHA could figure out a way to bring everyone together as a cohesive group. If I knew someone outside of my small area of control who was really good at something, I could get their resources and talk to them and feel more empowered. I think we're all just so disconnected. I know ASHA has those special interest groups. I wonder if some of that could be how to connect

RW: Any advice you would give to someone starting out in the field?

SLP: Reach out to people who've done it for a while to get some suggestions from them if you can find them. Just don't pigeonhole yourself into a certain area. Figure out what you really like.

I think we have to be diverse in how we approach kids and how we look at kids, and say, "This is how I'm going to get the best out of you." We have to be able to figure out what the child needs, and how we can get it to them. Until you can figure that out, I don't think you're all that effective.

RW: If you could go back to being an 18-19 year old, would you go back and do it again, or would you do something different?

SLP: I would go back and do it again because I honestly don't know what else I would do. You think about other professions, you meet people who are in other jobs, and you think, Well that sounds like an okay job, but I don't want to do that job. Honestly if I ever did anything else, I'd probably come back and be a PT or an OT, just because it's part of that therapy mindset, but I don't know if I would like it as much as speech.

I Have Absolutely No Regrets

RW: Why did you become a SLP? What drew you to the field?

SLP: My mom was a speech-language pathologist in Soviet Union. I grew up in Ukraine when it was part of Soviet Union. Obviously her work was very different from what we do now, the scope of practice was different, but I got introduced to the career as soon as I was able to walk and talk. She would bring me to work with her. She worked in a kindergarten that had services within that kindergarten. So it's very different, the systems are different. Basically any kid that attended kindergarten that the teachers, or she, thought might need help, she would just bring them to her office. No insurance. Not really any testing.

Even at the age of five and six, I felt like I was already supposed to supervise the children, so they would leave me on a playground to make sure all the other children were okay. Now that I think about it, this was so funny, but yes. So basically I wanted to work with kids myself since I was probably seven, and I knew that I wanted to do speech pathology. But my mom died when I was 12 and…

RW: Oh, I'm sorry.

SLP: I was kind of like, Okay, you're gonna do what you know. I loved it. I would work with kids. I was very zoned into something with kids. When we came to the United States I went into speech pathology, because I looked at the teaching, and I looked at the school systems, and I was like, I'm not going to be a teacher. The American educational system was very overwhelming in how it was done. So if that was a possibility in my other country, here it was not in my brain. So speech pathology was just a very clear course.

RW: What else might you have done if you weren't an SLP?

SLP: It's funny because I do think about it, what would you have done if you didn't know about speech therapy? There are many things I actually am into. I took a little break from speech pathology and went and got a master's in theater, mid-career. I'm also a stage manager and an arts administrator. It's a lot of fun. I actually find that the work is parallel. I mean, to be a good stage manager and a good art administrator, you have to be a good communicator. You have to know how to listen and you have to know how to look at the big picture, but also understand the details. I feel that if you're a competent SLP, you have those pieces, right? It goes hand in hand with the arts world.

RW: What have you found to be frustrating in our work?

SLP: For most of my career, I worked in early intervention, and that actually included working for the army. The last eight years have been my only time when I worked in a place that relied on billing insurance. I can tell you that one of the most frustrating things for me is when the insurance people decide what is appropriate for my clients. During COVID I was seeing as many kids as I could via telehealth. A lot of my kids were not appropriate for telehealth because their families just couldn't do it, there was too much going on. A lot of my families have multiple children. When they were all learning from home, they didn't have enough devices and enough supervision to also do therapy right with a two or three or four year old.

I had specifically this one child who was with me, and I used to see him every day before COVID. Mom was amazing and she was able to do telehealth. So we did telehealth, but it was really hard because he needed significant support. He still does. A parent can be wonderful, but the progress could still be minuscule, right? He needed prior insurance authorization every three months. After this initial three months with telehealth, insurance said, "Oh, he's regressing, he's not making any progress. So he doesn't need services twice a week. We're only gonna approve once a week." And I said, "In which common sense formula can you show me that a child is not making progress while we are living through a pandemic, something that most of us have not experienced before? It's an incredibly stressful time for everybody."

 We're literally just all looking for any support resource that we can find, and you're telling me that you're gonna cut services to this child. All of a sudden he's at home with just Mom and brother, a very loving home, but it's very different, right? All of a sudden he's home instead of coming to our program five days a week where it's four hours a day, where he was receiving mental health services, OT [occupational therapist], and speech and language, and just being in an environment with other peers. This is a child where I'm actually documenting home programming and where Mom is able to follow through. You're gonna tell me that he doesn't qualify for more than one half hour a week?

So that's just one story. But every time something like that happens, where the insurance blatantly says that they're not gonna cover something because "We just don't cover speech and language services," it's like, "Why do you not think that communication is an important part of a person's being?"

We needed to get an AAC [augmentative and alternative communication] evaluation for another kid. We work with an AAC company and thank God, somebody comes in, and she's really great. She helps us with insurance. She said, "Oh yeah, there are some insurance companies that will not cover an AAC device at all, unless a person had a laryngectomy." So those are the things that are incredibly puzzling. I can't even tell you that they're frustrating because they're so out of the realm of common sense and decency for me.

A lot of the doctors after an autism diagnosis will prescribe ABA [applied behavior analysis therapy], because insurance will pay for it, and because you can get it eight hours a day. We have a family that's leaving our day treatment next week, not because Mom is not happy with the services, but because Mom got a job and needs a place for her child.

RW: How do you get through that kind of frustration, how do you keep going?

SLP: I know that what I do and what my colleagues do is really impactful. I have done it in a variety of settings, and I know that we can't solve every problem. I know that we don't have enough services for everybody, right? So it's not necessarily that I'm closing my eyes to ABA [applied behavior analysis]. But also, to be honest, I don't believe in ABA. I don't support what they do. I think that it's traumatic and abusive. It's kind of like in ABA, they pretend they're SLPs. A lot of our families don't even know that they're not getting speech and language services. You have the CBA [certified behavior analyst] with maybe an undergraduate degree, maybe none at all, who goes in and pretends like they know what communication is. But I also understand that there are programs that call themselves ABA and they're really not, because they do work better than most ABA programs. If they work with older children and teenagers, they mostly work on functional skills, like how to use a microwave or how to go to a corner store and get a soda.

If children cannot go to an academic setting because there isn't enough support there, we just don't have programs that are not ABA that provide services.That's really frustrating to me. It's probably because insurance doesn't pay, and probably because there are ABA programs that a family sometimes needs as a kind of respite. During COVID, I don't know how some families survived having their children that require significant support at home, children that are older that are physically more able to hurt you.

 My hope is that as we keep talking about neurodiversity, and as we keep talking about how ABA is not good and is harmful, that there will be funding to develop programs that are not that restrictive and that don't do as much harm. Programs that actually focus on functional skills and the needs of the client. That's my hope. The frustrating factor is that there is no funding to do all of that. So that's the truth. I keep going because I know that they need it. All of my colleagues are doing wonderful work and there are many professionals that are amazing all over. That's what keeps me going, because I also see the impact.

I was doing home visiting, and what I really miss about that is communication with families. Sometimes that was frustrating too, because a lot of families didn't have resources. I've worked with a lot of them that didn't have enough money to buy food. I've had single moms that worked at night and they literally needed to take a nap when I was there. It's like, that's not how you do early intervention. But at the same time they will either not have me come, and the children will not get services at all, or they can rest and then I can do some coaching and we can provide some resources. I think that again, the black and white with a lot of our professions where you have to do this and this and this, that's not life and you have to think how it works for each family. You have families that walk away because they're too overwhelmed. That's really upsetting too, knowing that the family is not going to be getting services even though they need them because they can't handle one more thing.

RW: What else needs to change in our field?

SLP: Our field is so vast. I think depending on where you are, there are different things that need to change. For example, my paperwork is not that much, but I know if you talk to school people, they will probably tell you different things. Productivity. I feel like sometimes the mentality is, we need to see as many children as possible because we need to make money in order to keep our program open, and that's true. But if you overwhelm the people that work with you, they will burn out. And I found times in my career when I had no time to do any kind of home programming. I had no time to sit down and call a parent or a school teacher or a doctor, because my caseload didn't allow for that. We have to use cancellations and no shows to do the paperwork that we have.

Again, none of that is gonna change unless we get better funding, and maybe not through insurance. Maybe if there is more federal money to actually provide support services, then we can concentrate on meaningful work. I also think that we have some young SLPs that come out of grad schools with an idea of a cookie cutter. It takes a long time to learn, and maybe sometimes they don't, that it's not a cookie cutter and that you meet the family and a child where they're at.

RW: Do you have a favorite story?

SLP: This day treatment program that I've been working in for eight eight and a half years works mostly with families that are Somali refugees. We have families that have multiple children that are autistic, so we have families where multiple children come for services. I have one family that I've probably worked with for the last six years, and I work with all three children. The last time I saw the Mom, we were actually at a gala for our program where we tried to raise a lot of money, and she said, "I have adopted you into my family, so you can use my last name as your last name, because I know that I can always email you, or come and ask you things."

RW: Oh my God. I'm tearing up here. She gave you her name.

SLP: I'm not religious at all, you know, but she's more so. She said to me, "I pray for you every night because I don't know where me and my kids would be without you." Actually I've never considered our profession or myself as like a savior, because that's not what it is. What I want to do is to be there to empower our families so that they know how to advocate for their children. This mother is advocating for her children because she's using the resources that she knows, and she also knows to come back and ask questions. It's really touching when she says, "I pray for you."

All three of her sons are incredibly amazing. I love working with each of them, but I don't know how she single-parents them, because of the amount of energy that takes. I'm like, I don't understand how you're not laying on the floor. She goes to school to teach the peers of her older son who has autism how to play with him, because he doesn't know how to make friends yet. She goes during recess and plays with all the children to show them how they can play with him.

RW: That's phenomenal. Any other stories you'd like to share?

SLP: We had an OT that started working with us, and she went to some kind of CEU [continuing education unit]. We were in a team meeting and she said, "I just learned that kids with autism like men better than women, because they like their vocal quality better." I was thinking, What? What study was that? That was just something that was said in her CEU class. Then one of our speech therapists was told by an OT that a tongue tie affects your coordination.

RW: Your tongue coordination?

SLP: No, the coordination of your body. Like it will make you wobbly.

RW: (laughing) How is that possible?

SLP: The SLP was going on and on about this, and I was like, I don't understand. You know, people ask questions about tongue tie all the time, and the only research finding we have is that it can affect breastfeeding. I asked this SLP about the body coordination thing, and she said, "I wish I had the research. I don't. But I work with some really good OTs and this is what they told me. If someone had told me that a year ago, I would have thought it's bananas. But I have a lot of children with tongue ties that are completely different after surgery." I'm like, OK, I've got families that tell me their child got a vaccine and that's why they have autism. There are a lot of young therapists who are extremely impressionable, and will accept anything without much contemplation, and it's really hurting kids.

RW: Any advice for someone starting out in the field?

SLP: You know, I would have given myself this same advice though I know that I wouldn't have followed it. As much as I love early intervention and as much as I loved being very focused with EI, and now with autism, I also know that it's incredibly important to have a bigger worldview of our profession.

When I was in grad school, I didn't even do a school placement, even though I think I drove my graduate director nuts because I was the only one that basically said, "No I'm not doing a placement in a school." I said, "I will never work in a school. I promise you that," and she said, "You don't know," and I said, "No, I do. I will never work in a school." If I was that graduate director now, I probably really would not like myself, because I was a problem, right? She needed to find another early intervention placement for me because we did four placements in my grad school. I said, "I am going to do early intervention," and I did, and I loved it.

I think it would be beneficial to have a more open-minded kind of view, do a hospital placement or whatever. Our profession is so vast. Before I came here the youngest child I worked with was probably eight months old, and the oldest child I worked with was three and a half. Here we work with children up until they're 12 or 13. At first, I was like, oh my God, I need to learn things really fast. It's one thing to work with a kindergartener, but middle school, that is a very different world. It was later in my career, so I was fine, because I think that as you become more mature in what you do, you know how to get those resources and how to learn and figure out on your own. I guess my advice is to keep more of an open mind because you never know where your career is gonna lead you.

RW: If you could go back in time, would you still become an SLP?

SLP: I would. I love the kids and I love the families. The only thing I would do differently is learn to negotiate better. You do need money to live.

RW: Any regrets?

SLP: I have no regrets. I have absolutely no regrets.

Be Patient With Yourself

RW: What brought you to the field? What made you decide to be a speech therapist?

SLP: I've been asked this question over the years. I feel like they asked this question at every orientation, and I always felt like I had to kind of create a very meaningful, elaborate answer to it. I guess it wasn't anything in particular. I never had speech therapy as a kid. I didn't really know kids that had speech growing up. I was raised in a family with a heavy medical background; my mom's a nurse, my sister's a nurse, and my brother's a clinical lab scientist. I have dentists, doctors, all the allied health professions in my extended family. It's kind of always been an expectation growing up that I would do something in the medical field. But I never really felt like I fit in with what it was to be a medical professional. I didn't really feel I fit in that category.

My sister had a friend that became an SLP, and she kind of broke down the different populations you could work with for me. She said that there was a high need at the time, and it would be an easy transition from college to working. I was kind of just looking for a path that I knew would get me independent and on my own and stable, and that sounded like a good option at the time. So I just went with it, and I did it straight out of high school, straight through college.

RW: Was there ever anything else that you thought of becoming?

SLP: I was always interested in culinary stuff, just anything food related. I remember before I went to college, going to the Culinary Institute of America close to Napa, and taking a tour of the place to see if that was something I wanted to do. But the tuition there was $75,000 a year. There's no guarantee that you would get a return on that investment. That was before I knew how to research different programs, and what to look for. I was like, Oh, that's not an option, as a high schooler. I just kind of went with the option that was laid out in front of me and became an SLP.

RW: How are you feeling about it now?

SLP: That's a complex question. I would say it's going okay, it's going alright. I wouldn't say It's going fantastic, but I wouldn't say it's going horrible either. I started my first year out of grad school the year of the COVID shutdowns, so I only got about half a year to just get my feet wet in my first job in the schools. Then they shut down halfway through the year. I feel like I'm still catching up as a professional, and I almost feel like I've regressed a bit because of that year. When they mention all the time in school about learning loss from COVID, I feel like I was kind of robbed as well of having at least a whole full year of work to kind of get established and figure it out.

RW: That had to be really hard. I can't even imagine starting out in the middle of COVID, that's brutal. Is there anything about the field in particular that frustrates you?

SLP: I would say I feel a bit isolated on the job. Day-to-day, there's not really any other professional that understands what we do as far as the school system goes. It's like all the other teachers kind of just know you as the speech teacher. I'm trying to imagine how SLPs look to them from the outside. It's kind of tough to do that. I think it's definitely an isolating feeling, being the only one of your profession on the job site.

RW: For sure. Is there anything else that frustrates you so far?

SLP: My caseload this year is not as bad as my first job. My very first position was also in the schools. I was a contract company employee. I was kind of naive taking a contract position in the schools my first year, because I didn't consider that contract jobs are paid hourly and not salary. If you consider the schedule, as a contractor you have unpaid weeks off at a time throughout the year for vacations, and then you're left with only a third of a paycheck. It just doesn't really make sense to take a school contract job. I don't know how people do that. I was on a single income at that time, so I had to figure it out or put things on credit to get by.

Something else that was frustrating was the caseload of that first job. There were 75 kids, and a lot of them were kids that looking back now didn't need speech therapy for what they were working on. I had to do a lot of cleanup as far as whether they actually needed to be receiving speech therapy, and if so, how much. I basically had to rework the whole caseload at my first job, and I had no idea what I was doing. But it was a good learning experience.

RW: For sure, it was learning how to make those clinical decisions as to who really qualifies and who doesn't. What do you find rewarding? What keeps you going in the field?

SLP: I would say just kind of being a part of my students' lives, being able to enrich them, where I can, and seeing the effect that has potentially on their family dynamic. Just kind of being a little piece of the puzzle.

I am pretty introverted, so I don't like being publicly recognized for helping if that makes sense. I'm not a fan of that attention. It sounds so silly when I say it out loud, because as an introvert I didn't consider a career called speech-language pathology would make me exhausted by talking. It's not really something that clicked until I started working.

RW: Until you actually live the experience of doing something, you don't know how it's going to impact you.

SLP: Right, and I feel like a lot of SLPs on average are very bubbly and out there. I don't really have that personality. I'm also seeing that affect me as a team member as well, coming into this. This is also my first year working in the elementary population, and with preschool. My first three years were in secondary, middle and high school. I feel like elementary SLPs especially are known for being bubbly and extroverted, and just really high energy. I'm more of a listener and synthesizer when it comes to my style. I can tell that my other staff members were kind of expecting a big bubbly personality, and it seems almost like it's a bit of a disappointment that I'm not like that. It's never been spoken out loud. It could be my own insecurities about it, but It's definitely something that I've intuitively have been feeling a bit.

RW: I'm sorry, because that's really unfair. I think that everybody brings their own personality to the table and that's valuable. Have you felt any burnout so far?

SLP: I kind of ebb and flow with burnout. I have some weeks where I'm feeling pretty good about it, it's steady. And then there are months that are just super heavy paperwork and meetings. What really burns me out are IEP meetings. I feel like they tire me out, especially if I'm the case manager, because it just means that I'm gonna be the one talking and coordinating and discussing everything for half an hour to an hour straight. By the time I'm done with three IEPs, I just want to sit in my office and do nothing.

RW: I think it's draining.

SLP: See, it's interesting that I ended up in the schools, because during grad school, I was way more interested in the medical courses. I was also an anatomy teaching assistant for two years.

RW: Wow, that's impressive! Do you think about making a move into the medical aspect of speech?

SLP: Definitely. I feel like I kind of just settled for the schools starting out, but that's just what's more readily available and in your face when you finish grad school. All the contract companies and school districts, they're all searching for staff, and they will go to job fairs. It was just an easier option to start out knowing that I would have something lined up after I finished school. Now that I've been doing this for a few years, I feel like I'm trying to make the schools work for me. At the same time, each year I feel more and more that I don't know for sure if this is the right population or setting for me. There are parts of being a school SLP, like having the school schedule and being salaried, which are big perks. But the job itself, I don't know if it's fulfilling to me. I feel like I might transition into home health, or telehealth.

RW: From what you've seen so far, what needs to change in our field?

SLP: I feel like at a national level SLPs are underpaid on average. You can always find high paying SLP jobs, but they are few and far between. I would also say because our field is so broad there should be an option to specialize in grad school so people are more prepared when they start their jobs.There's so much within our scope of practice that I feel like there's no way possible for a grad student to feel at all prepared. When you start your CF [clinical fellowship] year, in any setting, there's definitely not enough to fully prepare you, and I feel like that's a little scary. At least you do have a CF supervisor to kind of guide you, but CF supervising can be hit or miss as well. If you get a not so hands-on supervisor, you're kind of shit out of luck, I guess.

Something else I wish would change, but it's kind of like a snowball at this point, is that there's a lot of SLP influencers popping up, starting specialized training programs that aren't vetted by any organization necessarily. They might be loosely evidence-based, or not really evidence-based at all, and they're selling a specialized course. It's kind of just leaching money off of other SLPs in a way. I don't know what should change about that, but I think it's not a great look for any medical profession.

RW: Do you have a favorite SLP story?

SLP: I have a story from my first job in a middle school setting. I was working with a kid in a severely handicapped classroom. He finally got one sound that he had never been able to say. When he finally got it one session, he just had the biggest look in his eyes, and he kept saying it. He was just so excited. Then he told his mom about it, and the mom called me and was really happy. I guess it was kind of like my first family moment working with a kid.

There are plenty of crazy stories, though, as far as IEP meetings go. I had a case last year where there were no longer academic concerns, but the kid previously had some speech goals. I was the case manager. The demands from the kid's grandmother were just so high, and she basically lost her mind and started screaming at the principal and interrupting everyone, not allowing anyone else to speak. That went on for like 20 minutes straight. I'm just here trying to seriously take notes of everything everyone is saying, while grandma is telling me what I should write in my notes. That was one of my toughest IEPs. There have been others where the family has a lawyer and the kid has 30 IEP goals, and every little word is picked apart. I think I had one of those meetings with another family that lasted three hours, and that's almost half the work day. It was exhausting and demoralizing.

RW: What has been different from what you might have expected?

SLP: I think I kind of romanticized it a bit as far as, "Oh I have so many options to do all these different things." Which I do, but at the same time it's not always realistic to to shift gears into all the different parts of the field on a whim. You really gotta commit to a job, if you're going to do it. At least starting out, you've got to start with something and stick with it and figure it out.

 RW: What advice would you give to someone who was thinking about becoming a speech therapist? Any words of wisdom?

SLP: I would say, "Take grad school with a grain of salt, it's not gonna prepare you for everything, and that's okay." When I first started I was so stressed with 75 kids on my caseload. I asked my CF supervisor, "When does this job start making sense? When did you feel like you had kind of a grasp of the field?" This is my fourth year, and as far as the day-to-day operations of being an SLP, I feel like that's starting to make more sense, just because it's something I've done for a few years. Now it's just starting to become a routine part of the job, rather than stressful. I would say be patient with yourself. Give yourself that time to really figure out the job. Whatever area of the field you choose, it's okay to not know everything.

RW: Would you do it all again? Any regrets?.

SLP: I wouldn't say I regret it. I think the people I've met and the things I've learned are overall good things. That being said, I don't know if I would necessarily do it again. Getting to know myself over the past eight years of doing grad school and then getting into the field, I've been learning more about myself being an introverted person. There probably would have been a field that suited that part of me better and would maybe have fulfilled me a bit more. I'm also young and I've only been in one setting, so that could always change.

Boots on the Ground

RW: Tell me about your experience in the field.

SLP: I started out in 1993 wanting to work with adults. I've got to tell you that I'm probably not a great person to be questioning, only because even when I was in graduate school, I knew that this was really not for me, but I continued on because I just wanted to finish what I started. At this point I would really love to transition out of the field completely. I'm not sure I can do that, but I'm going to try.

I used to read the *ASHA Leader*. I would look in the back at the employment ads, and I can remember at least once, if not twice, that I was able to locate my next employer there. There were private agencies and private school districts hiring. The job search section was so much bigger back when we graduated, but within the last 10 or 15 years all of these middle-man companies have just scooped up all that work. I hate the fact that you don't talk to or deal with the actual school district. Talking to the contract companies, it's "I'll take the money and run," versus "I'll hate it," because mainly the school districts that you're paired with are just absolutely a mess

My goal out of school was to work in rehab with adults. But gradually over the years, my clients got younger and younger. After I finished my CFY, I went to work at a special education school. But because I had never gotten the teaching credentials to work in the public school system, because my original intention was not to work with kids, I worked mainly in the non-public /private sector. A lot of my work has been in the area of private practice. It was a little bit challenging at times. Right now, I'm working in early intervention, that's probably my favorite setting or situation of all, really. It's been nice.

RW: What are you thinking you might do if you leave this field?

SLP: I was a freelancer a few years back in a couple of local papers, but again, I wasn't earning enough to really keep it going. Then I published in a couple of online magazines, *Autism Parenting* magazine was one. I kind of would like to keep pushing myself to do freelancing. But as far as a real job, that's a really good question. I've even talked to job coaches and career coaches, and just still don't have a clear idea other than having to go back to school and incur even more debt, and I can't do that. I'm just trying to explore something that would allow me to use my writing to create. Instructional design is not totally totally off the table, or instructional writing.

RW: What initially drew you to the field?

SLP: What attracted me initially was thinking about being a teacher, but I didn't want to deal with a whole classroom of kids. I wasn't sure at the time whether or not Adult Ed would be an open door for me. I wanted to be able to teach, but I wanted to be able to do it in small groups, or maybe even one at a time. I ended up choosing speech therapy by an indirect route.

A regret that I have is not pursuing instructional design. I went to grad school originally not to do speech, but to do instructional design. But unfortunately, there was a lot of emphasis on the tech part of it. I thought, Wait a minute, where does my teaching come in? I wish I had stuck it out a little bit more, but I was a kid in my 20s and I was ready to throw it over. I didn't want to give myself enough of a luxury of time to really sit back, just get a job, and say, "Hey, what do you really want to do?" To be honest with you, I felt very pressured. So, I chose the speech department and I was accepted, and that's kind of where I ended up. I wanted to do something that involved a bit more creativity, that maybe didn't involve dealing with groups of people, and had an element of education or teaching in it.

RW: Can you talk about what frustrates you as an SLP?

SLP: I feel like we don't really get paid enough. I'm sure you've heard this before. We get paid, but we don't get paid enough to really comfortably support ourselves, despite a master's degree. I hate to say this: A lot of us are do-gooders. Many of us I've met are overachievers, who if you tell them to jump, will say, "How high?". That's great, but there's a flip side. We get exploited because we're such hard workers and such dedicated souls. We don't want to let anybody down, and we don't want to leave our clients out in the cold. So we do the right thing, always.

RW: Do you think that's related to the fact that most of us are women?

SLP: Absolutely. We're people pleasers, we're women. You and I might be about the same age. We supposedly grew up in those "liberated" 70s. Well guess what? It wasn't very liberating. We were still raised to do certain kinds of jobs which are still seen as quintessentially female jobs. We're thought to have husbands who are supporting us, and this is all a vanity project for us, instead of some of us having to support ourselves and our kids.

I felt very put down in graduate school. I didn't struggle per se, but I guess maybe partly because I wasn't totally buying the project, or wasn't totally into it, I wasn't as dedicated as some of my fellow students. I was just kind of phoning it in, I hate to say. I felt a lot of disdain from a lot of other students. I think there was a lot of intolerance for differences, even of opinion. Mistakes were not cool, asking questions would not be cool. It was just very childish and it felt very much like being with a group of mean girls, and you just couldn't get away from them to save your life. The professors and supervisors didn't really help. So you go on not really wanting to ask questions, but in the back of your mind thinking, I'm not really buying into this, and made to feel like you're just very incompetent.

I've felt that since that time in various jobs that I've held. I can't seem to escape it. But I say to myself, "You know what, this was never your dream, and whatever cognitive or mental space you gave it, you did your best. And you know you'd better be off somewhere else. You've known that for a very very long time. So all things considered you've done pretty okay."

RW: Absolutely. Do you relate to the concept of imposter syndrome? Because a lot of SLPs that I'm talking to can relate to that.

SLP: Boy. It's weird. Yes, I'm going to agree with that. You can check me off and put me down for that. Speaking to how I felt when I went to school and maybe my state of mind then, I didn't feel like I was very well prepared to actually do therapy. In the back of my mind I'm thinking that it would be really cool to be able to talk to someone about this, but feeling like I wasn't able to do that. Somehow we were just supposed to sort of divine doing therapy from watching maybe a few people do it. So it's a combination of that, and of the field being broad, and feeling certain programs or situations did not prepare you realistically for the job in any way whatsoever. You're left feeling like you're supposed to be an "expert," when in fact, what they need to tell you is that it's going to take you maybe three to five years before you start to really feel comfortable, and that's if you're staying at the same job and not switching gears every couple of years.

So much of our clinical information is behind a paywall that some of us are ashamed to say we can't handle financially. Maybe you're working part-time, or you're working as a contractor, or have your own business, you've got to drum up the money to get trained in something new, training that we don't get in graduate school. We should be getting it in graduate school. Dysphagia is an example. I'm sorry, one class ain't gonna cut it.

RW: What's kept you going?

SLP: What's kept me going is the fact that I have a family. I've had to keep doing this. I live in a rural area, and so other job opportunities may be out there, but they're very far away. When my kids were younger I worked part-time and I was able to be there for them. There was convenience to it, though it was financially difficult. The hours were flexible, so it was a situation that I didn't want to give up. I figured this is my training, this is what I do.

Even that presented some problems. I ended up having some health problems, and when my boys were sick, there were times when I didn't want to just bring them in to work with me and leave them in the TV room there. That job was a match made in hell, and they ended up letting me go. It was really ugly and I wish I had retaliated, but I didn't at the time. I was kind of relieved to be away from them. It was just a really unpleasant experience. It was a situation, again, where I've had to keep going because of finances.

I've tried different settings too. I have left several jobs, and I only allow myself to tell another SLP that by adding that my tolerance for things that don't work out has absolutely plummeted. I can tell if this is not for me, and I'm not going to waste anyone's time or my time, so I'm just going to say "Thank you very much for the opportunity. But on I go."

RW: That's wise. Have you had some rewarding experiences?

SLP: What I liked when I was a student was creating my own learning materials. That kind of stepped into the instructional designer that might still be in me. I don't have the energy in private practice to see child after child, seven or whatever hours in a row, five days a week, so I try to do it part-time. I'm doing evals, mainly. I'm not doing any real treatment, only maybe one or two, but I like the kids. I like their families. I like the idea of really helping them to access services. There were things about it that I did like, but to be honest, I just didn't like doing therapy.

The sweet part of my job is just dealing with kids and grateful parents. I've had the luck of being with families who feel like whatever it was that I had to offer, whether it was an evaluation that was comprehensive in their mind, some tips and tricks, guidance, or saying, "Hey, you guys got this. Don't worry." That's the best part for me.

RW: If you had a magic wand and could change anything in the field, what would be different?

SLP: I would revamp the standards of what qualifies an SLP nationwide so you don't have these differences between programs. I would also make sure that training or courses in school were reevaluated, and perhaps updated, maybe every two or three years. I don't know what kind of an overhaul that would be, it might be very difficult, but I would really want that as far as EBP [evidence-based practice]. We want to make sure that we're keeping current. For example, the whole idea of neurodiversity needs to be really brought in with a vengeance. You've got to present that to people right off the bat.

Quite frankly, I would unionize us in some way. I guess that different parts of the country have different costs of living, but at the very least, we should all be earning something commensurate as a base salary. There needs to be caps on caseloads regardless of setting. The gig working, all that crap, that needs to go. We have to have some sort of protection, even if we're part-time, even if we're contracted. Maybe that's where a union can help us out.

I also think ASHA is smart to create the mentor program. We need to have more mentors. We need to be each other's best friends. I feel we need to stick together, we need to have each other's back. I am no longer on Reddit but when I was reading the SLP Reddit I would see a lot of comments about mentorship. There's been a lot of comments about needing to really just dive in and try to change this field from the inside, and maybe even try to do it by joining with ASHA. I'm a little jaded. I kind of get the feeling they collect our dues and they offer us maybe some discounts, and they tell us what the standards are, but beyond that I feel like ASHA doesn't really advocate for us.

RW: What advice do you have for someone entering the field?

SLP: I guess if a young person came to me today and said, "You know, I'm thinking about going into speech and language therapy," what I would tell them depends on where they choose to be. I would fill them in on everything, and I would encourage them to consider a setting that would give them the benefits and the pay, like working for a school district or maybe working for the VA [Veterans Administration]. If you're okay with those settings, I would say go ahead, because you're going to pay a lot in student loans. A lot of our work is done in somewhat precarious settings that either attempt to compromise our ethics or practices, or pretty much work us into the ground, and don't really compensate or offer us much in the way of benefits.

I see speech therapy as being part of the largest systems, and I think those largest systems are failing us. If you work in the school, look at how many teachers now supposedly are quitting the field. If you're in the medical area, you're working with our messed up healthcare system, at least speaking only of the United States. We're just part of a larger web, and we're feeling the crunch, because we are so close to the ground with the public. We are the boots on the ground.

Take Care Of Yourself

RW: What drew you to the field?

SLP: I actually wanted to be a nurse. As a kid I was volunteering as a candy striper and I love the medical field. I started as an eighth grader, and then in high school all the nurses said to me, "Do not be a nurse. There's no respect. The nurses are dumped on. They're treated poorly." All the nurses that I became friendly with would say, "Don't become a nurse." So then I thought, Oh, maybe X-ray or something in the medical field, because my mother worked at the hospital. She was a single mom, divorced, and my dad was really not in the picture, so she was also working a second job with an ENT who was a family friend. So he said, "What about audiology?" and I went, "I don't know what that is." He said, "Look into audiology or speech pathology." Well, audiology did not interest me one bit, but speech pathology sounded really good, because I knew I wanted to do something with kids. So I looked into it and here I am.

RW: What frustrates you about our field and your experiences in it?

SLP: What frustrates me is the micromanaging behaviors of the administration, who really don't understand what we do, how we do things, and why we do things. They really don't understand no matter how much in-services or materials you give them. The micromanaging, and the unrealistic expectations of the amount of kids you have to see in the amount of time you have. It's just, "Group them together and see them. Well, I don't care if he's on the spectrum and is working on communication skills, and the other child is an AP student who stutters." They just want the numbers, instead of really letting us do what's good for the kids. It's not good for anybody. It's not.

RW: So what keeps you going anyway, despite all the frustration?

SLP: Well, I retired in June, and then I went to work for an agency. I've been back working in the schools. I really didn't take off any time before I went back with the agencies, but it's really refreshing, because I don't have to get tangled up in the school politics. I don't have to deal with parents that are unrealistic. The agencies are just so happy to have me because their therapists were on leave. Next week, after spring break, I go to another district who's desperate, and so they're willing to do whatever. I'm like, "I'm taking a bunch of vacation," and they're like, "Whatever you can give us!" So I see how I was treated before as a district employee. It's far different from being a consultant. They love to have you.

So what keeps me going, I guess, is I love what I do. I love seeing the gains that the kids make, I love the relationships, I love helping the teachers to help the kids. It fills this chronic need of me to be a people pleaser and heal-the-world kind of person. What's rewarding is when you can help a student to understand their disability, so that they can figure out what strategies they need to be successful. Working in high schools was really rewarding when kids were told by guidance counselors or administrators, "You can't do this, you can't do that." Then I get them in my office saying, "Don't listen to them. This is how you could do it."

I'll never forget, I was at a wake and this man in a suit sees me. He runs up calling my name, and he picks me up and spins me around! I looked at him, and he said, "Thank you. I am so glad you're here. I would never have made it to be a state trooper without you.That was my dream, to be in law enforcement, and they told me I couldn't do it because I couldn't think fast enough."

RW: That's so beautiful. You empowered him.

SLP: Right. Another kid was told he could never survive as a chef in culinary school. I told them, "Don't listen to them," and they wound up graduating from the Culinary Institute of America. When they say they can't, you just show them a different way to do things. "You'll figure it out, if you want to do it bad enough. There's people there to help you, take advantage of it."

I remember that first student I had at the high school on an AAC [augmentative alternative communication device]. It was the one that would print out the tape that looked like a cash register receipt. I will never forget him. He had cerebral palsy, you couldn't really understand anything he said, so he used a device with the head switch. This was all new to me, because it was just new AAC technology.

The teachers would just dismiss him.They would only ask him for one word answers. I had him in my office one day, and I told him, " Merry Christmas." Then I added, "I know we're not really allowed to bring God into the public schools." He typed in, "Please wait." He started switching away, and gave me a dissertation on how the separation of church and state is good. He just went on a roll of telling me what he thought, and then he told me he wanted to become a minister.

 I thought, Nobody's ever given this kid the time, because it took probably the whole 40 minutes I had with him. But what he wrote to me with that device, using his head to operate the switch, blew me away. And I went back and I showed it to every single teacher. I said, "You're treating him like he's a kindergartener and he's a 16 year old guy who has a brain that's filled with wonderful thoughts and ideas.

RW: I love that! On a different note, what needs to change in our field?

SLP: I think we really need to teach the schools that we can't bring every kid in for speech. I see all of these kids with lisps that have no other impact other than they sound different. Yes, they do have something wrong with their speech or their sounds, but it's not affecting them academically or even socially. Some of these kids feel great about their speech. Yet, we're still seeing them because we feel like we should fix them, or the school says we have to see them. Some of these kids don't belong here, they need to be in private therapy, so I think we really need to have some kind of connection with private therapists.

There's this disconnect. I have 50 kids at this new school for speedy speech, that's five minute speech. I see 50 kids a day for five minutes each, not to mention the regular groups and the other things I'm doing. It's insane. I keep saying to the teacher, "Well, how's their spelling? How's their reading? How's their writing?" They say, "Oh, fine." Well, then why are they here? I've brought this up so many times, but schools are afraid that if we give recommendations to private therapists, we're saying that they need therapy, and then the school is responsible for paying for it. So I think that's clogging up the caseload.

On the other end are the parents who have the most severely disabled kids who are really not going to get really any better. I had one child last year, he was in a wheelchair, major spine issues, nonverbal, barely attentive. He couldn't even turn his head on his own, and they had him for speech two days a week. This is a high school kid in diapers, tube fed, private nurse. Mom thinks he's gonna talk, and wants him in speech therapy five days a week for an hour a day, and the district didn't want to fight her. He functions at a six months old level. It's tragic, but what are you gonna do? That's where he's at cognitively. So you tie up a therapist just trying to get him to maybe turn his head to a sound source.

RW: What advice do you have for someone who's starting out in the field?

SLP: Take care of yourself. Look for ideas and resources that you could use for a variety of populations, like finding materials that you can adapt in many different ways. But definitely take care of yourself. Do not let them suck the life out of you.

I think for the new people, I just look at them and they are so eager. I'm supervising somebody who's finishing her clinical fellow year. She actually took my old job which I retired from. She just started last month, and she seems so timid, and so fearful. I keep saying, "Don't be afraid to make a mistake, you're not gonna kill a child, we're not tube feeding, these kids aren't gonna aspirate on us, not this population. So just have fun."

RW: Do you have any regrets? Would you do it all again?

SLP: I would do it all again. I would definitely do it all again. No regrets, but maybe what I would have done differently is stand up more for my needs in the public schools, really let them know this room is insufficient, and so are these materials. In my attempt to be accommodating and flexible, I was stepped on. Looking back, I should have just been a little bit more like, "No, I'm not gonna take that, or I'm not gonna do that."

You Wouldn't Ask Your Dermatologist…

RW: What drew you to the field?

SLP: A crisis in college of not knowing what I was going to do. I went to college as a physics major originally and very quickly realized that area of science wasn't for me at the time. It's a ton of really hard classes, you're in a new place, all you want to do is go and have fun with your friends, but you need to be at class at 8:00. Then you're like, well, if I'm not gonna do this, then what am I gonna study? I was going through that book of all the majors and I came across communication disorders. My grandfather had pretty significant hearing loss, so I had some familiarity with audiology. I read a little bit more about it, and thought, "This sounds really interesting to me, why don't I take the introductory course and see," and I just went with it.

I was always a helper. I'm still a helper, and I think that's really why it connected with me, because the field really is about helping others and making connections. I think that's what kind of drew me in and had me keep going.

RW: What else might you have liked to do besides speech?

SLP: When I was in high school I wanted to be a baker. I still love baking, but thinking about the logistics, their job is not just, "Oh I get to bake today!" It's really a lot more challenging than it is if you're just a hobby baker. I double majored in psychology. Perhaps I might have still gone into therapy, but more on the mental health side of things. I also think if I had known about occupational therapy at the time when I learned about speech therapy, I might have also gone that path. I have much more of a math brain than a language brain.

RW: When you look at the field and think about your experiences in it, what would you say you find frustrating?

SLP: I could probably talk to you for days and days about what frustrates me about this field. I was really trying to think, what do all of these things that frustrate me have in common? What does it stem from? And what I came up with boils down to the fact that our scope of practice is so immensely huge and vague. There is so little public education about the field. I was even talking to a good friend yesterday, and she has no idea what I do. She just thinks that I either work with little kids that are developing or not developing language, or fixing sounds. So you know public perception of what we do is just so limited, and yet our scope is so vast.

I really see a lack of valuing us from the public and from healthcare, and a lack of appreciation. You can really see it in insurance reimbursement rates and what Medicare has us paid. They are continually cutting rates. Ok, If I work with a specific diagnosis, they value me, but I don't think health care or the educational system as a whole really values the therapists that work for them, because they really don't know what we do or how we add value. Those things really lead to reduced quality of care across the board. That is really what frustrates me. Our scope is so huge, and education amongst the public is so limited that it just creates barriers.

RW: What else would you like to see change in the field?

SLP: It's kind of like a double-edged sword here, but I would really love to see a model that mirrors how doctors specialize. They go to med school and then they can specialize and have fellowships in different areas. Having so many areas really requires speech pathologists to be generalists, but then they are really discouraged from referring to therapists that have chosen to specialize or have more competency in some areas. I would love the field to really embrace specialization, because when you get therapists who are so much more confident in specific areas, the quality of care in those areas really increases. You wouldn't ask your dermatologist about your vision problems, right? So why would you ask your AAC therapist about your stuttering problem? I do think specialization can also create a barrier to accessing care, so it's kind of a balance of how we would move in that way without really putting lots of people's careers in jeopardy.

I'm nine or so years into my career. Earlier on I had imposter syndrome every single day. Now I specialize, and some days, I feel so confident that absolutely what I'm doing is working. Other days I'm just like, Oh my God, why do I ask people to give me money? I think those feelings are really resolved for myself when I consult and provide a lot more parent and caregiver education. I see people in their homes, so their families are in our sessions.

But what sparks that imposter syndrome for me in those situations is if I'm thinking about what they're seeing. What they're seeing is me, following around their child, who doesn't look engaged at all. I'm just modeling on a device, right? I'm thinking, This doesn't look like anything. So it's in those more challenging cases, where really all I'm doing is trying to be able to connect with their child and model language in a way that they are not used to, that I feel imposter syndrome. I think the family is looking at it and not understanding what I'm doing. So it's important when I can provide that education and explain why it looks like we're doing nothing, or when I tell them to model and say, I know it feels like you're doing nothing, but you are.

RW: What keeps you going then?

SLP: I have such strong connections with my clients. Earlier out of my career, I was really looking for those big gains. Did we meet the goals? Now what really keeps me going is those small incremental changes, although those are really huge steps, at least for the people that I'm working with. I work with children and young adults who have really complex communication disorders. I specialize in augmentative and alternative communication. So for me, and for parents, some gains might seem really small, but for the people that I'm working with, those small gains really are huge. Being a part of those changes and having those connections with my clients is really what gets me up in the morning and keeps me slogging through all the things that I hate doing.

Another thing that keeps me going is when my clients are finally able to access and use language for self-advocacy. So many therapists aren't comfortable with AAC, but they want to use it anyway. They're locked into just working on this requesting skill, right? I come in and I'm like, we need so much more language. There are so many more reasons to communicate than saying, " I want Goldfish."

I have a teenage client, and when I came in not even a year ago, she had a device that she wasn't using at home. She was hiding it under the furniture, and when you looked at it, it was so limited. It only had vocabulary on there that she could use at school, and it's basically for answering yes/no questions or requesting food or games that they have available. Now we've gotten her a device that has robust language, thousands of words, and we're slowly modeling using it. She still needs help navigating the screens, and I had navigated to a page that had some comments on it. She told me, "Bye, bye, I don't want to work on this!" and I just said, "Okay, bye!" It's so great that she can tell me that! She's 17, and she hasn't had access to language like that before. I'm thinking, I'm so sorry that you're having a hard day and you don't want me to be here, but at the same time I was just so happy that she's able to express that. I have a lot of stories like that where someone hasn't had access. Sometimes it's that parents want their kids to go with the flow, and be compliant, and just to make life easy for them. I just love it when my clients can finally say, "I don't want to!"

RW: What advice would you give to someone who's just starting out?

SLP: I think it is to observe as many different therapists in as many different areas of the field that you possibly can. I know that that's more challenging than I would like it to be, but I think the reason so many of the people that are finding out that they don't want to be in this field at all is because they really didn't know what they were getting into. Talk to as many SLPs and observe as many as possible before you sign up for it.

RW: Did you know what it was going to be like when you started in the field?

SLP: My undergraduate university had a clinic, and that's where I got all of my observation hours in. I got a very narrow view of what therapy was gonna look like. You can read about all of the different settings, but when you actually observe what's happening, observing grad students giving therapy is very different from observing skilled, experienced clinicians giving therapy. And so no, I don't think in undergrad I understood really what my day-to-day was gonna look like.

My day-to-day work doesn't look like sitting at a table and doing very structured activities anymore like it did at a time when I worked in a clinic setting or when I worked in the schools for a couple years.That was a different experience, because now my day-to-day is very natural functional based therapy. It's a lot more modeling. I didn't really get to observe any of that, and it's taken me a really long time to understand how to change therapy to suit different types of people. I love what I do now. I didn't like working in the schools, but I was able to separate the field itself from working in the school setting.

RW: What was it about the schools that you didn't like?

SLP: Often you're in a district that piles on your caseload and doesn't value you, encourages you to work longer hours than you contracted to, and doesn't give you enough resources and time. It's impossible to do your job in the school setting, although there are some exceptions. There are some smaller school districts that really value you, and don't give high caseloads. The vast majority of people that work in schools are overworked and underpaid. I didn't last very long in the schools, but that didn't really color my whole view of the field, right? I knew what I wanted to do and I just needed to get out of that setting.

RW: Do you have any regrets about becoming a speech therapist?

SLP: I think my only regret is my really high student loan debt. I went out of state for undergrad, and grad school is so competitive that I only got into one school, and it was a private school. That was another $100,000 that I had to take out in loans. I graduated from grad school in 2013. It's been 10 years, and my student loans are higher than what they were when I left. I make a decent living, but those loans are gonna be with me until I'm 50.

The unfortunate thing for those of us who took out such a vast amount of student loans is that loan forgiveness isn't really going to help. I'm not gonna feel it. It's gonna help so many people who have smaller amounts of loans. But not for someone like me who's riding out an income based timeline, where I'm trying to make minimum monthly payments for 25 years. Only then my loans will get forgiven, and I'll be paying income tax on all those payments, right? So, I'm not gonna feel it if $20,000 gets forgiven today. I'm all for it for the people it will help, but it's not going to help those of us with really high amounts.

When you have this dream, "I just want to go to school, I just want to become this," you think, "I'll worry about loans later." You don't think about a high number like $150,000 plus interest when facing your dream. There's no one there to tell you what it looks like down the line.

RW: So would you do it again?

SLP: I probably would apply to different schools if I could do it over again, but maintain my knowledge. I would probably do things differently so that I didn't have as many student loans, but I would go into this career again.

RW: Is there anything else you'd like to add?

SLP: We need to get on board with this neurodiversity movement. I've really evolved and changed the way that I practice in the last couple of years.The more autistic SLPs and autistic adults that we can learn from, the more support we can be for those individuals.

You're My Family, Too

RW: What brought you to the field?

SLP: Basically the same thing that almost didn't bring me to the field, my mom's a speech pathologist, and I didn't want to follow in her footsteps. So I went to school as a psychology major thinking I'm going to be a child psychologist, like half the rest of the world thinks. But I actually didn't want to go to school forever, and psychology is just too long.

My mom worked at Easter Seals when I was a kid. At that time, it was called the Crippled Children's Center, which is kind of sad. I grew up volunteering in the preschool classroom and working with all the kiddos, and falling in love with them. That's kind of what I knew and I liked it.

RW: In looking at your work, what would you say frustrates you?

SLP: My biggest frustration is that people don't look at speech therapy as valuable, or even as therapy. There's a lack of understanding. They don't understand what we do. Part of that's our fault for being called speech pathologists, and they're wondering, "What is that?" I come in and the patient's always saying, "I'm waiting for therapy." I say, "I'm from therapy," and they respond, "Oh no, I want to walk." Well, you're not just a pair of legs, and it would help if you knew not to walk in front of a bus. It's not just the patients and their families, it's the other people at work, the other professionals. They just don't get it. Even insurance companies. They'll say, "Oh, they can walk a hundred feet. They can go home." But they might burn their house down because of cognitive issues. It's just that lack of understanding and a lack of desire to understand.

They think we're just not important. People will come to the nursing home with an aspiration pneumonia diagnosis, or with altered mental status, and they don't have speech orders. How is that a thing? I always ask the nurses and the aids, "How's Mrs. So-and-so?" and they're like, "Oh, she's eating fine, and she can talk." But does she know what the hell she's saying? They just don't get it.

Once the family of my patient's roommate brought my patient peanut butter crackers. She couldn't have that, she couldn't swallow it. They were going to kill her. When I explained that, they just looked at me, and then they said, "Do you have to go to school to do this?" I don't mean to be disrespectful, this sounds really horrible because I love the nurses' aids and couldn't do my job without them by any means, but I thought, "Well, I wanted to become an aid, but it was too much education, so I became a speech pathologist instead." I was so mad.They were awful.

RW: What about the field keeps you going?

SLP: It's helping the patients and the families, and the relationships that you build, and seeing progress. Seeing them be able to return to their lives, which sadly doesn't always happen. Or helping family members get through tough times. I feel like half of our job is counseling. I think we should have gotten more classes about that. I remember taking a class about counseling parents of exceptional children, but I don't remember any other counseling-based classes and I feel like we should have had more.

RW: Do you have a favorite story?

SLP: I had a patient who oddly ended up dying of pancreatic cancer, which is what my first husband died of. She was cognitively 100%, she was all there mentally, but physically she was a mess. She had to walk with a walker with somebody standing by her, she had a tracheostomy, and she had a fused spine. She also had arthritis and did not have good mobility or dexterity, and her larynx was basically anchored, so it couldn't move up and forward. She always sucked on candy, even though she aspirated everything. She couldn't tolerate a Passy-Muir Valve [speaking valve] at all.

I started seeing her after a hospital stay. We got her able to wear the speaking valve. The catch was since she couldn't physically take it off, she had to be around people when she had it on. She couldn't qualify for an augmentative device, but we did get her the speaking valve, and she was just a force. Her first swallow study that we did indicated that she could only tolerate carbonated liquids, and that was it, but she wanted tomato soup. So I was getting tonic water and mixing it with soup. It was pretty disgusting, but that's what she wanted.

She ended up getting up to a mechanical soft diet with thin liquids. We were actually in an article in the paper that showed us with our little frappuccinos from McDonald's, and it was really neat. She was a bit of a high maintenance lady, but I told her I would always have her back, so whatever weird things she'd ask for, even when she wasn't on my caseload, I'd say, "You just call me." She was the sweetest. Everybody loved her.

And then she ended up with cancer. I remember when she came back to the nursing home from the hospital, basically to die. I went in, and her family was there, and I said, "Well, I'm gonna let you be with your family," and she said, "You are my family. You are my family, too." I just loved that woman so much. I said, "I'll come back to see you tomorrow." She died that night.

RW: Such a beautiful story. What advice would you give to someone entering the field?

SLP: When I had a student I gave advice that I don't use myself necessarily. Make sure that when people read your report, that it stands alone so they don't have to look through the chart for more information. The one thing that I always slack on, that everybody else does too, is when you're supposed to document about medications and interactions you don't put anything. I was trying to be a better example for my student. Technically, we want someone to be able to just read your report and not have to look at anything else.

I remember in graduate school when I did an internship at an intense rehab hospital. I would feel really guilty about what I was able to do that they weren't. I had a teenager who dove off a building into a swimming pool, and he'd done it a million times. But one time, he hit the bottom of the pool, and had a pretty high spinal cord injury. He had a trach, and was on a vent [ventilator]. I'd be water skiing and I'd think about him. I felt guilty, but you can't do that. We can't really leave it at work, but you have to try at least to separate yourself. Appreciate what you can offer them, but don't beat yourself up because you have abilities that they don't, or resources that they don't. You just can't save the world. You've got to be able to be a healthy human in mind, too. It's like we tell the families, take care of you, because if not you won't be able to take care of your family. If you're not taking care of yourself, you'll be in the next bed. So we should listen to what we tell our families.

RW: Would you go back into it all again?

SLP: I think so. If I think about what else I would do, I don't feel like there's anything else that I connect with. I have a lot of new interests that I didn't have when I was a kid and I certainly have broadened my horizons, but I still think that I'm in the right place.

RW: And so you have no regrets?

SLP: I wish I would have done better in school and in my internships. I think I kind of sucked back then, but I think I've learned. I think it's a learning curve.

Author's note: I went to school with this SLP. She didn't suck. Not even a little.

Printed in Great Britain
by Amazon

23846634R00069